ANALYTIC METHODS
—— in ——
Maternal and Child Health

The material in this workbook was developed initially for:
DEAL MCH: Enhanced Analytic Skills Program
(DHHS/PHS/HRSA/MCHB)   (MCU-17D501-03-2)

Arden Handler, DrPH
Principal Investigator & Core Faculty

Deborah Rosenberg, PhD, MS
Core Faculty & Co-Project Director

Joan Kennelly, RN, MPH
Core Faculty & Co-Project Director

Colleen Monahan, DC, MPH
Core Faculty

This workbook is published in collaboration with:
MCH-Info: Analytic Software Tool for Needs Assessment
(DHHS/PHS/HRSA/MCHB)   (MCJ-17D601-03-0)

Colleen Monahan, DC, MPH
Principal Investigator

Division of Science, Education, and Analysis
Health Resources and Services Administration–Maternal and Child Health Bureau

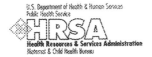

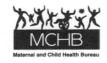

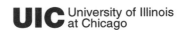

Production Coordinator: Margaret M. Maloney
Desktop: Wendi Thourson & Christopher Tedin
Cover Design & Graphs: Jason Millet

Published May 1998

For information about *Analytic Methods in Maternal and Child Health* or the electronic version of this book, please contact:

Arden Handler, DrPH		Colleen Monahan, DC, MPH
The University of Illinois at Chicago		The University of Illinois at Chicago
School of Public Health	or	Division of Specialized Care for Children
Community Health Sciences		Research and Development
312.996.5954		312.996.1360

Copies of this book are also available from:

The National Maternal and Child Health Clearinghouse (NMCHC)
2070 Chain Bridge Road, Suite 450
Vienna, VA 22182-2536
703-821-8955
nmchc@circsol.com

Module 6: Creating Target Population Estimates Using National Survey Data 233
Colleen Monahan, DC, MPH

Module 7: Using Census Data in MCH 257
Colleen Monahan, DC, MPH

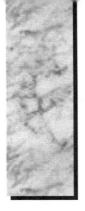

Preface

This workbook is an outgrowth of efforts by the University of Illinois School of Public Health (DEAL-MCH and the MCH Training Program) over the last seven years to develop and implement a training program to enhance the analytic skills of maternal and child health professionals in state health agencies. In its seven offerings, this program went through many iterations and in each provided a variety of different analytic modules which attempted to capture the skills needed by those involved in MCH assessment, planning, evaluation and policy development. Unfortunately, we cannot include all of these modules in this workbook. Those included offer new perspectives or insights to traditional topics (e.g., epidemiology, biostatistics) or offer fresh material that specifically addresses applied analytic issues confronted by MCH professionals in their daily work (e.g., summarizing data).

In producing this workbook we have teamed up with our colleagues from *MCH-Info: An Analytic Software Tool* project so that we can provide an electronic version of these modules as well as a print version. We are hoping that the availability of the material in two versions will facilitate its use as a training tool, self-instruction guide, and general reference.

We encourage you not only to read the basic text but to actively participate in learning by completing the Test Yourself questions and the Exercises and reading the accompanying Answers and Solutions which elaborate on the material found in the narrative. Similarly, the *Comments and Examples* sections offer either a different perspective or additional detail that complements the main body of the text. While it is not necessary to read the modules in order, or in particular, to read the epidemiology-biostatistics modules before the others, the usefulness of the workbook as a training tool or self-instruction guide may be enhanced for some individuals by working through the material in the order presented.

We look forward to your feedback as you use this workbook.

Acknowledgements

This workbook is the result of the efforts of the many faculty and staff who participated in the Enhanced Analytic Skills Program (EASP) over its 7 years. We would like to acknowledge all of them here.

EASP Staff
Manu Khare, MS
Kendra Phillips, MPH
Rita Ruhter
Mary Kate Weber, MPH

EASP Guest Lecturers

Catherine Alter, PhD, MSW
Jill Anderson, MSN
Bernard Baum, PhD
Don Blose, MS
Laura Brey, MS
Noel Chavez, PhD, RD
Kathleen Crittenden, PhD
Kevin Croke, PhD
Faith Davis, PhD
Alan Dever, PhD, MT
Timothy Dye, MPA, PhD
Richard Ferguson, MSPH
William Hollinshead, MD, MPH
Vijaya Hogan, DrPH
Sylvia Furner, MPH, PhD
Matthew Johnsen, PhD
Tim Johnson, PhD
Michele Kelley, MSW, ScD
Russell Kirby, PhD
Kathy Knafl, PhD
Frederick Kviz, PhD
Cara Krulewitch, PhD, RN, SNM
Katherine Kvale, PhD
Claudia Lampmann, PhD
Patrick Lenihan, MUPP

Cathy Melvin, PhD
Ed Mensah, PhD
Katie Merrell
Margaret McManus, MHS
Geraldine Oliva, MD, MPH
Magda Peck, ScD
John Peterson, MD, MAPA
Kendra Phillips, RN, MPH
Karen Quinn, PhD
Viswanathan Ramakrishnan, PhD
Janet Reis, PhD
Linda Remy, PhD
Kathleen Rhodes
Mary Rogers, DrPH
Roger Rochat, MD, MPH
Erica Salem, MPH
Susan Scrimshaw, PhD
Sharon Telleen, PhD
Bernard Turnock, MD, MPH
Kathryn Vedder, MD, MPH
Barbara Waggoner, MPH
Gayle Winston
Martha Wojtowycz, PhD
Tisha Dowe-Westmoreland, MD, MPH
Terri Wright, MPH

Some help with the technical aspects of the trend module was provided by Sally Freels, PhD, V. Ramakrishnan, PhD and Laura Schieve, PhD. James Hagen, PhD provided assistance in developing exercises for the epidemiology and biostatistics modules. Sally Freels, PhD and Sylvia Furner PhD provided thoughtful comments on the epidemiology and biostatistics modules.

Last, we also want to acknowledge two very special people without whom this effort would never have been possible, Naomi Morris, MD, MPH who initially applied for funding from the Maternal and Child Health Bureau to develop an enhanced analytic training program at the University of Illinois School of Public Health and Tom Loesch, educational consultant, who introduced us to competency based education and who gave us the tools that allowed us to share our knowledge and skills with all of you.

Enhancing Analytic Capacity in State Health Agencies through Competency-Based Education:

Observations of the Enhanced Analytic Skills Training Program at the University of Illinois School of Public Health

by Arden Handler, DrPH

INTRODUCTION

Since the publication of the Institute of Medicine's seminal report, *The Future of Public Health* (IOM, 1988), public health agencies have been enhancing their capacity to more effectively carry out the three core functions of public health: assessment, policy development, and assurance. Support for enhancing public health agency capacity has been undertaken at the federal level by the Health Resources and Services Administration (HRSA) and the Centers for Disease Control and Prevention (CDC) of the Department of Health and Human Services (DHHS). These agencies have increasingly turned to schools of public health for the creation of new models of continuing education and professional development designed to enhance the analytic capacity of state and local health agency staff. The goal has been to increase the ability of state and local health departments to engage in information based decision-making.

In 1990, the Maternal and Child Health Training Program of the University of Illinois School of Public Health (UIC-SPH) received a grant from the Maternal and Child Health Bureau (MCHB) of HRSA to develop and implement the Enhanced Analytic Skills Program (EASP), a continuing education program for practicing Maternal and Child Health (MCH) professionals. This was one of four grants given to schools of public health to assist state health agencies to enhance their analytic capacity through either changes in the masters or doctoral programs in MCH or through continuing education programs. The Maternal and Child Health Bureau's effort to increase the analytic focus and skills of MCH professionals was a response not only to *The Future of Public Health* but also to the Omnibus Budget Reconciliation Act (OBRA) of 1989 (Public Law 101-239) which mandated new data analysis and reporting requirements for Maternal and Child Health Block Grant recipients in state health agencies.

The Enhanced Analytic Skills Program at the University of Illinois was designed to improve the analytic skills of MCH professionals in state health agencies. National in scope, EASP served 93 MCH professionals from 44 states and three territories in seven separate offerings between 1991 and 1997. Its educational premise was competency-based education, which utilizes methods in which participants acquire skills and knowledge that directly enable them to better perform their tasks and responsibilities in the workplace; the acquisition of knowledge divorced from application is antithetical to this approach.

Competency-Based Education

A competency-based educational approach was chosen because it is thought to be best suited to adult learners participating in continuing education programs (Harris, et al., 1995). Competency-based education requires: specification of learning objectives in behavioral terms; establishment of criteria by which to assess individual achievement of competencies; provision of instruction that is directly relevant to the learning objectives; and, assessment of the learner's ultimate experience with respect to the established competency criteria (Elam, 1971; Houston and Howsam, 1972). Therefore, UIC-SPH Maternal and Child Health faculty and staff worked together with educational consultants to develop a curriculum that would be rooted in the day-to-day experience of MCH practice, be "hands-on" in approach with a focus on real problems and issues faced in the workplace, and which allowed for the assessment of achievement of competency at regular intervals throughout the program as well as after the program's completion.

At the time of the establishment of EASP, the competency-based approach was just emerging as a viable educational strategy for training professionals in schools of public health (Public Health Faculty/Agency Forum, 1991). With an increasing emphasis on public health practice as the basis for learning, the development of the EASP curriculum demanded an entirely new orientation for the UIC-SPH faculty involved. Armed with the understanding that even familiar content would have to be organized and presented differently, EASP faculty were challenged to identify and assess the functions performed by state level MCH professionals and to translate these into a set of skill-based modules.

Defining the Competencies Needed by Maternal and Child Health Professionals in State Health Agencies

The development of the EASP curriculum began with the delineation of five key activities of state-level MCH staff: surveillance and monitoring, needs assessment, program planning and administration, program evaluation, and policy development. The next task of the planners was to review the skills and knowledge that were necessary to perform each activity related to these functions. Seven competency areas were identified:

1. The ability to develop primary data-sets;
2. The ability to utilize secondary data-sets;
3. The ability to conduct statistical analyses;
4. The ability to use computer systems and packages;
5. The ability to conduct needs assessments;
6. The ability to develop program evaluation and research designs; and,
7. The ability to develop and maintain quality assurance, monitoring, tracking, and management information systems.

For each skill area, the tasks necessary to develop and demonstrate competence were translated into learning objectives, which were then used to direct the content and learning methods of each module. Emphasizing real data, case problems, simulations, and group problem solving activities while minimizing the traditional lecture format, EASP modules mimicked the participants' work environment to the extent possible, and promoted an interdisciplinary team approach to public health leadership and practice.

The Evolution of the EASP Curriculum

The initial EASP curriculum was developed just as states were beginning to struggle with the data requirements set forth in OBRA 1989, and before many state health agencies had begun to switch from a focus on the delivery of personal health services to a more core function, population-based approach. The curriculum was adapted over time to meet the needs of MCH programs and the rapidly changing environment in state health agencies. Modifications to expected competencies, learning objectives, and module content were based on participant feedback and evaluation of each EASP offering, a growing understanding of the needs and expectations with regard to the level and kind of analytic activities assumed to be appropriate for state MCH professionals, and the acceleration in technology and its increasing availability to state health agencies. While some curricular changes were also related to time and resource constraints, the majority were made in an effort to develop a program that was directly relevant to the needs of state MCH professionals, particularly as states made the transition from a clinical services delivery approach to a population-based approach to meeting the needs of women, children and families.

Observations Gleaned from Enhanced Analytic Skills Training for MCH Professionals in State Health Agencies

The fundamental assumption underlying any analytic skills training program in MCH is that the ability to effectively collect, analyze, and report data will directly lead to the design and implementation of effective programs and the development of appropriate policies to improve the health status of women, infants, children and adolescents. In attempting to meet the challenges of this assumption, during the seven offerings of EASP, we continually forced ourselves to reconsider choices in curriculum design, format, objectives and content. Curricular decisions were based on a number of intersecting factors: expedience and resource constraints, areas of faculty expertise, new insights on how best to mix and match conceptual and skill building components within and across modules, and the need to provide opportunity for practice and synthesis of course material, enabling participants to achieve the greatest degree of competency. Through our experience with the EASP program, we have made a number of observations about competency-based education for MCH professionals in state health agencies. These are offered here for others who are considering similar training efforts.

What is the appropriate format for competency-based enhanced analytic skills training for state MCH professionals?

Competency-based education requires demonstration, practice, and reinforcement of newly acquired skills and knowledge. In choosing an appropriate format for competency-based training to increase the analytic skills of MCH professionals in state health agencies, there are clearly a variety of options available, such as the short workshop or a series of short workshops, the intensive institute (greater than 3 days), computer-based distance learning, or a program which takes place over an extended time period and which incorporates multiple formats; each option is associated with different resource demands as well as different possibilities for learning. Clearly, not all of these formats allow for the same level of integration of substantive knowledge and skills; as such, when planning enhanced analytic skills training there needs to be a consideration of the tradeoffs of time, resources, and the intensity of the learning experience. Within time and resource constraints, the format should be selected based on its potential to allow participants to sufficiently absorb, integrate and translate their newly acquired skills into their daily activities in the workplace.

In making a decision about format, it is also important to consider the role of peer and colleague interaction in the learning experience. When participants are engaged in a group learning situation over an extended period of time, the opportunity increases for interchange and learning from peers both within and outside the classroom setting. Although there is always danger of exhaustion or overload, there seems to be a minimal amount of time (at least 3 full days) required before the benefits of this interaction really begin to manifest. In fact, it appears that this interaction is maximized when participants have at least one week of consecutive time together.

Sufficient time also needs to be built into the training to allow participants to engage in activities and exercises in the direct presence of instructors, so that issues and concerns are immediately addressed. Without such opportunities, participants who return to demanding work schedules, may feel less confident in using their new skills in the home setting, and in some cases, will be reluctant to do so, or will not be able to do so with a great degree of ease, comfort, and confidence. Even when EASP was offered as a two week session, with a break between weeks, there seemed to be a need for more time to adequately practice skills, suggesting that a format which also includes ongoing support or mentoring by the instructors may be optimal. Most importantly, participants need to be provided with the opportunity and support to use and sharpen their newly acquired skills in their home states.

Who should be trained in a competency-based enhanced analytic skills program for state MCH professionals?

Enhancing analytic capacity within state health agencies requires a commitment by states to the role of information-based decision-making in program planning, management and policy development and a concomitant commitment to increase the analytic skills of staff involved in these activities. As MCH programs in state health agencies shift their focus to population-based activities and as the demand for accountability increases for all programs, it will likely be necessary for the analytic skills of all MCH professionals in state health agencies to be augmented to one degree or another. Therefore, enhancing capacity in state MCH programs requires two strategies. The first strategy is the hiring and/or (re)training of staff specifically dedicated to performing analytic activities which support and promote information based decision-making for maternal and child health. Depending on the organizational structure of the state health agency, these individuals may be located within the MCH program or within adjacent units such as vital records, or in related agencies, such as the state Medicaid program. A second strategy for enhancing capacity requires increasing the ability of those MCH staff whose primary focus is not analytic work to articulate their data and information needs when interacting with their more heavily focused analytic colleagues.

The EASP program's initial offerings focused on enhancing the capacity of MCH administrative and program staff to better understand and express their data and information needs, and to increase their ability to collect and utilize data to address MCH problems. However, over time, the program increasingly focused on meeting the needs of a newly emerging cadre of data analysts in the states, whether these individuals were newly hired or had been recently transferred into new positions. These individuals, while usually possessing basic analytic skills, were not necessarily trained in applied methods, or if newly hired, needed assistance in translating their knowledge and skills to the MCH and public health agency setting. In addition, individuals whose previous job functions had been more clinically based, needed increased preparation for, and orientation to, a population based approach.

As state health agencies move to a more core functions based approach, striking a balance between enhancing the analytic skills of "program" staff and designated "analytic" staff should become easier. In this process, it is essential to move away from job titles to job functions and to ensure that analytic skills training is provided to all those whose daily activities focus on some aspect of the data cycle at a level appropriate to their efforts and responsibilities. While EASP training emphasized the need for an interdisciplinary team of individuals with a variety of skills working together to increase the analytic capacity of the state MCH program, our effort also recognized that analytic skills training needs to occur at multiple levels. EASP chose to fill the particular niche of advanced training because this type of training permits participants to return to their states as leaders capable of moving the analytic efforts of their agencies forward. This "train the trainer" approach, allows analytic skills training to reach a greater number of individuals in state health agencies, while simultaneously promoting the development of MCH state data leaders.

How should competency be assessed in a competency-based enhanced analytic skills program for state MCH professionals?

As skills are being developed during the course of analytic training, it is necessary for participants to practice and demonstrate competency with respect to these newly acquired or enhanced skills. There are a variety of methods to accomplish this; these include variants on traditional formats such as tests, essays or papers, or the use of exercises/practice sessions or interactive case scenarios. Exercises, either narrowly focused on the mastery of a particular skill, or interactive case scenarios which bring together a variety of exercises, allow participants the best opportunity to practice what they have learned as well as demonstrate their mastery of these skills. When utilizing the case scenario approach, it is possible to develop independent cases to accompany specific modules or to use one or two unifying cases in which aspects of the case situation are directly related to several modules, with skills learned in a previous module necessary to complete the next part of the scenario. The use of the unifying case scenario allows for greater synthesis and integration of knowledge and skills than the use of independent cases or exercises, although this may not be the best approach when the program has a short time-frame or very specific skills are the focus.

How much hands-on knowledge of computers is necessary in a competency-based enhanced analytic skills program for state MCH professionals?

When we began EASP, learning analytic skills in conjunction with the use of the personal computer was not seen as essential. In fact, participants submitted data requests to EASP faculty who then conducted appropriate statistical analyses using a mainframe computer. This process was in essence "mimicking" the typical vital records-MCH staff relationship assumed to be prevalent in state health agencies in the early 1990's. However, as developments in technology accelerated and as health departments began to avail themselves of this increasingly user-friendly technology to conduct analyses with a variety of data-sets, it became clear that while not essential, analytic training would be strengthened by incorporating the use of computers. Using personal computers (laptop computers can be rented for a reasonable cost for an extended period) in the curriculum provides participants with hands-on experience with both user-friendly analytic software readily available to state health agencies (e.g., Epi-Info, Epi-Map) and with new analytic methods or techniques. It also provides participants with the opportunity to practice their newly developing or enhanced analytic skills in a way that they typically find very engaging, and enables them to return home with clearly "visible" skills.

What content and skill areas should be included in a competency based enhanced analytic skills program for state MCH professionals?

While the curriculum in the initial offerings of EASP attempted to address the seven competency areas delineated above, it became clear that some of these competency areas needed to be emphasized over others (e.g., ability to develop and maintain quality assurance, monitoring, tracking, and management information systems was deemed to be such a major, complex and specialized focus that it was excluded from the EASP program) and that some (e.g., ability to develop primary data-sets) were really building blocks in achieving more fundamental competencies such as the ability to conduct a needs assessment. Over time the curriculum solidified around the following elements which we suggest are essential to effective enhanced MCH analytic skills training:

1) **Information Based Decision-Making as Foundation:** An appreciation of information-based decision-making in public health as an essential first step to developing and enhancing analytic capacity should be a fundamental premise of analytic skills training. As part of this foundation, a discussion of the definitions of health and public health, an understanding of the statutory authority and role of public health, and an appreciation for the philosophical underpinnings and underlying

assumptions which anchor public health policies at the national, state and local levels can be incorporated. Anchoring public health decision-making in an understanding of the interplay between public values, popular opinions, and the level of our scientific knowledge is essential.

2) **Planning Cycle Functions Framework:** The analytic activities engaged in by MCH professionals in state health agencies revolve around the planning cycle: surveillance, needs assessment, program planning, program monitoring and evaluation, and policy development. Presentation of a strong conceptual framework which focuses on the components of the planning cycle is therefore a necessary underpinning for analytic training in MCH. Without such a foundation, newly acquired skills are less likely to be successfully integrated into an individual's skill and knowledge base and are less likely to be appropriately implemented in the participant's work environment.

3) **Epidemiology and Biostatistics as Building Blocks:** Epidemiology and biostatistics are scientific tools for public health and the essential building blocks for advanced analytic modules. Without a requisite understanding of their basic principles, analytic skills training will not be successful. While enhanced analytic training requires individuals to possess some knowledge in these areas before participation in training, a review of the basics of biostatistics and epidemiology before proceeding to advanced topics strengthens participants' confidence in their existing skill and knowledge base. However, relevance to practicing MCH professionals requires emphasis on the application of these tools in the practice rather than the research setting.

4) **Advanced Skill Areas:** Analytic training programs must be on the pulse of emerging issues which are essential to the analytic work of analytic professionals in Maternal and Child Health. Curricula should be revised as appropriate to both expand and fine tune skill areas for development. Examples of content areas which were developed into EASP modules to meet emerging demands for increased competency include: systems analysis, economic analysis, analysis of trend data, summarizing data for decision-making, small area analysis and geographic information systems, and population based program evaluation. Of note, each one of these offerings required several iterations as understanding the importance of a skill or substantive area was not always easily translated into effective educational modules for practicing MCH professionals. As future enhanced analytic skills training programs emerge, an assessment of new areas in which competency needs to be enhanced is necessary.

5) **Key Data-sets:** Incorporating didactic and practice sessions using data-sets which are of increasing importance to the analytic efforts of MCH professionals in state health agencies is an essential component of enhanced analytic skills training. At various times, EASP modules were offered which focused on the use of hospital discharge data, census data, Medicaid claims data, the Child Health Interview survey, and the National Maternal and Infant Health survey, while traditional data-sets such as vital records continued to form the basis of many exercises. When incorporating these data-sets into an analytic skills training program, the extent and level of interaction with the data will vary depending on time and other resource constraints; however, participants should be familiar with the purposes, strengths and limitations of each particular data-set. The goal is to promote creative and maximal use of available data-sets to answer and address questions and concerns relevant to the maternal and child population.

Within the limitations of time and available funding, operationalizing and combining all of these elements into a successful analytic skills training program requires an appropriate balance of didactic presentations, skill building sessions, practice exercises, and individual assessment in order to engage and sustain participants as they develop and enhance their analytic skills. Achieving this balance always involves trade-offs and an understanding that each training program or offering cannot meet the multitude of training needs of state level MCH professionals. While recognizing that the "perfect" training program does not exist, incorporating some or most of the components described above provides an empirical foundation on which to base the efforts of future MCH analytic training programs.

THE MODULES IN THIS WORKBOOK

The modules in this workbook reflect the effort of the last seven years and the contribution of all of the faculty of EASP. While the majority of EASP modules are not included, we believe that the modules which do appear here contribute new information or new insights that are not found in a similar format elsewhere. In keeping with EASP philosophy and practice, we have incorporated examples and exercises throughout the modules so that the user of this workbook can learn at their own pace or with their colleagues, testing themselves as they proceed. Alternatively, the workbook can be used as a reference manual to which an MCH professional can turn to check or review an analytic approach. The workbook assumes that the user has had some previous exposure to graduate level epidemiology and biostatistics.

We share this workbook with you, our MCH colleagues engaged in information-based decision-making so that we may reach those professionals who applied to EASP, but who we were not able to serve, as well as the many other individuals whose job responsibilities are changing as their health departments begin to de-emphasize the delivery of personal health services and focus on the core functions of public health. It is our hope that this workbook will contribute to the ongoing effort to increase the analytic capability within state and local MCH programs to improve the health of women, infants, children and adolescents throughout the nation.

References

Elam, S. *Performance Based Teacher Education: What is the State of the Art?* Washington, D.C: American Association of Colleges of Teacher Education, 1971.

Harris, R., Guthrie, H., Hobart, B. and Lundberg, D. *Competency-based Education and Training: Between a Rock and a Whirlpool.* South Melbourne, Australia: Macmillan Education Australia PTY, LTD, 1995.

Houston, W. and Howsam, R. *Competency Based Teacher Education: Progress, Problems and Prospects.* Chicago: Science Research Association, 1972.

Institute of Medicine, Committee for the Study of Public Health/Division of Health Care Services. *The Future of Public Health.* Washington, D.C.: National Academy Press, 1988.

The Public Health Faculty/Agency Forum. *Linking Graduate Education and Practice, Final Report.* Sorensen, A. and Bialek, R., eds. Bureau of Health Professions, Health Resources and Services Administration and Public Health Practice Program Office, Centers for Disease Control, 1991.

Epidemiology and Biostatistics
Modules 1, 2, and 3

Introduction

Epidemiology and statistics permeate the work of practicing maternal and child health (MCH) professionals today. Every time numbers or rates are reported, every time a statement is made comparing numbers or rates of one group to those of another, every time a program is designed to change the conditions giving rise to the numbers and rates, the principles of epidemiology and statistics are being applied.

Often, however, the application of epidemiologic and statistical concepts remains at the intuitive level because standard textbooks and professional training materials rarely address analytic issues in the particular forms encountered in practice. Typically, these subjects are presented in the context of research, focusing on medical risk factors and outcomes or, in the language of epidemiology, on exposures and diseases. The core functions of public health, however, situate the work of MCH and other public health professionals in a much broader context that calls for the synthesis of epidemiologic and statistical principles with those from health services research, evaluation research, economics, and other related disciplines.

The goal of these three modules is to more explicitly connect epidemiologic and statistical methods and concepts to the work of those who collect, analyze, and report maternal and child health data. Our experience with analytic skills training has shown that this seemingly subtle shift in perspective is in fact crucial for enhancing the capacity of MCH professionals to consciously and creatively apply epidemiology and statistics to the development of programs and policies that will improve the health of women, infants, and children.

In a complex and dynamic environment, statistical theory provides the basis for making estimates, assessing their accuracy, and formally testing hypotheses. The general rules defined by statistical theory provide boundaries within which reasonable and useful conclusions can be drawn. Epidemiology gives shape to the rules of statistics, adding specific principles for analyzing and interpreting patterns of health and disease in human populations. Epidemiologic concepts provide a framework for collecting and organizing the data that is most appropriate and relevant for answering the substantive questions in maternal and child health. These concepts guide the definition of populations of interest, the construction of meaningful samples, the selection of appropriate indicators, and the analysis of the relationship between risk and protective factors, and health outcomes.

These three modules are not intended as a comprehensive course in epidemiology or statistics. In fact, familiarity with basic epidemiologic and statistical concepts as they are typically presented is assumed. The narrative, examples, and exercises included here present epidemiologic and statistical concepts with a focus on their specific application to MCH public health data analysis.

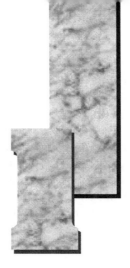

Descriptive Epidemiology and Statistical Estimation

by Deborah Rosenberg, PhD and Arden Handler, DrPH

EPIDEMIOLOGIC CONCEPTS

Epidemiology is the study of the distribution and determinants of disease, injury, and other health outcomes in human populations. Unlike clinical medicine, which focuses on improving the health of one individual at a time, the goal of epidemiologic analysis is to improve the health of the population as a whole. Of course, if the health of the population is improved so is that of individuals, but only with population data can the relationships between risk or protective factors and health outcomes be fully described and quantified. Moreover, a population focus shifts attention toward the role of public health programs and policies.

Typically, epidemiology is divided into two components: descriptive epidemiology and analytic epidemiology. *Descriptive epidemiology* focuses on identifying and reporting both the pattern and frequency of health events in a population; *analytic epidemiology* focuses on the search for the determinants of health outcomes. These two components work together to increase our understanding of the health of a population. The figure below shows the usual cycle of epidemiologic analysis:

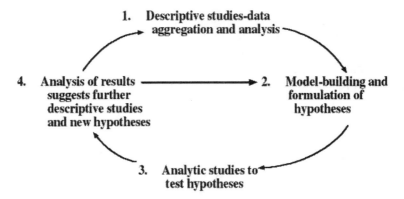

From <u>Epidemiology: An Introductory Text, 2nd Edition</u>, Judith S. Mausner, MD, MPH and Shira Kramer, PhD, Copyright ©1985 by W. B. Saunders Company. Used by permission of W. B. Saunders Company.

3

This cyclic process is at work in maternal and child health (MCH) when we conduct an analytic study based on the descriptive information obtained through surveillance and monitoring activities or needs assessments. Likewise, when analytic work identifies a new risk factor, we incorporate this new variable into our surveillance and monitoring activities. For example, as analytic research showed evidence of a relationship between smoking and alcohol consumption during pregnancy and adverse birth outcomes, these risk factors were added to the birth certificate in order to include them in routine surveillance activities. Similarly, the descriptive reporting of unintentional and intentional injuries spurred analytic work that led to the understanding of violence as a public health problem and the identification of risk and protective factors for the development of effective intervention strategies.

PERSON, PLACE, AND TIME

Descriptive epidemiology focuses on both the pattern of health events as well as on their frequency in populations. Within the field of epidemiology, there are three types of data that are necessary for describing the patterns of health and disease in human populations. These three pillars of descriptive epidemiologic analysis are:

1. Person
2. Place
3. Time

Person characteristics include sociodemographic characteristics such as age, race/ethnicity, education, income, insurance status, occupation, parity, and marital status as well as behaviors such as substance abuse, diet, sexual activity or use of health care services. *Place characteristics* include geographic location (e.g., urban versus rural), features of the geography (e.g., mountainous region, area with wells as the major water source), population density, as well geo-political boundaries (e.g., census tracts, cities, counties, or states), and location of worksites, schools, and health facilities. *Time characteristics* include cyclical changes, long term secular trends, and even daily or hourly occurrences during an epidemic. While person characteristics are attributes of individuals, place and time characteristics are attributes of the physical and social environment.

Another group of variables reflects the intersection of person characteristics with place and time. These *person-place-time* variables are person characteristics expressed in units of geography and time. Examples of this type of variable include the annual crime rate in a city, the extent of neighborhood segregation during a given time period, and the percent of low-income individuals living in a county during a given year.

By jointly considering person, place, and time, epidemiology advances the idea that health and disease result from the interaction between individuals and their environment. While we can all list various person, place and time characteristics without much effort, it is important to understand what these characteristics actually represent so that we use them appropriately.

Person Characteristics

Person characteristics are fundamental to describing health events. They are used to describe whether a particular risk factor or outcome is more prevalent in one population than another, or to describe whether the relationship between a risk factor and an outcome is more salient for one population than another. When using person characteristics to describe health events there are some issues that need to be considered.

Risk Factors vs. Risk Markers

Often by virtue of their strong association with an outcome, some person characteristics are themselves considered to be demographic risk factors. For example, the Institute of Medicine's report, *Preventing Low Birthweight* lists five demographic risk factors for low birth weight (LBW): age, race (black), low socioeconomic status, being unmarried and having a low level of education.

While lists of this type are commonly found, most of the variables they include are not risk factors but are simply risk markers. A *risk factor* directly increases the risk of a health outcome, implying a causal link; a *risk marker* is associated with a health outcome with no assumption of causality. Only if a person characteristic is an actual determinant of a health outcome, is it truly a risk factor. Otherwise, it is merely a risk marker, acting as a proxy for another variable, because this other variable is either unavailable in the data-set or is yet to be discovered or confirmed as a risk factor.

Public health professionals often confuse these two terms, with variables such as race or ethnicity being presented as risk factors when they may only be risk markers, representing some other underlying factor yet to be uncovered (e.g., stress, residential segregation). Occasionally, race/ethnicity is a true risk factor as in the case of Jewish ancestry and Tay-Sachs disease, or Mediterranean ancestry and sickle cell disease. When considering person variables, therefore, it is essential to think critically about the mechanisms through which these variables may be associated with the outcomes under study and to ascertain whether the variable of interest is a risk marker or truly a risk factor. This distinction is not merely a matter of semantics. The way in which variables are labeled can influence analysis and reporting strategies, which can lead to false conclusions about the relationship between person characteristics and health status outcomes.

Defining and Categorizing Person Characteristics in MCH

While it is important to understand the meaning of person variables, it is also important to be knowledgeable about the meaning of the boundaries used to define categories within the variable. What categories of the variable were used to collect the data and/or describe the data? For example, does the category "unmarried women" include women who were divorced or widowed as well as those who were never married? Does the category "adolescents" include 18 and 19 year olds along with youth less than 15 years of age? It is important to choose appropriate definitions and categories for the variables under consideration so that our efforts are grounded in the current knowledge base with respect to the variable(s) of interest and so that our findings can be compared with others who are doing similar work. Some key person variables used in MCH are described below.

Maternal Age. Maternal age is not a straightforward variable. The effect of a woman's age may represent operative genetic phenomena. A classic example of this is the association between Down's syndrome and increasing maternal age. On the other hand, the increased risk of an outcome associated with a particular maternal age group may represent the effect of the environment; exposure to a teratogenic agent at certain ages, for instance, can result in an increased risk of adverse outcome. Alternatively, an age effect may represent the interaction of genetics and the environment; for example, maternal age in conjunction with differential use of diagnostic technology and induced abortion may contribute to higher prevalence of genetic or chromosomal abnormalities for certain age groups. An association with maternal age may also be indirect, reflecting the impact of other factors such as parity, rather than a direct effect of maternal age itself.

Child Age. When describing the occurrence of health events in children, the focus is usually on age groups that are considered to represent distinct biological, social and/or developmental periods of growth and behavior, such as less than one year, or 15-17 years. Sometimes there is uncertainty as to whether a child's age places them at risk for a particular outcome because of biological or non-biological processes and sometimes there is interaction between these two phenomena. Again, while the tendency may be to assume that the age categories for children represent primarily biological processes, it is likely that understanding the social and development processes associated with these distinct age groups is as, if not more, important.

Race/Ethnicity. Race and ethnicity are associated with major differences in exposure to risk factors, in health service utilization, and in health status. While the way in which race/ethnicity variables are used often implies direct causal links between skin color or heritage and health status outcomes, race/ethnicity variables, except in a very few instances, are representative of social, economic or community processes or factors. It is usually more appropriate, therefore, to consider these variables as risk markers rather than risk factors. As the Centers for Disease Control and Prevention has stated in its monograph *From Data to Action: CDC's Public Health Surveillance for Women, Infants, and Children*, "The designation of race and ethnicity is often problematic, and definitions may vary from one data collection activity to another. Race is frequently a marker for a variety of cultural, economic, and medical factors, and these factors must be taken into account when assessing the effects of race on health outcomes."

Parity. *Parity*—the total number of viable pregnancies, including live births and fetal deaths—and the related variables of prior reproductive outcome and birth order are all associated with maternal, infant and child health status. Knowledge of these variables is important because:

1. the outcome of one pregnancy tends to be repeated in the next;
2. a prior pregnancy outcome may affect the mother's current status vis a vis work or schooling; and,
3. behaviors or conditions present in one pregnancy may be repeated in the next.

Of note, the association of higher parity with adverse pregnancy outcomes may not be a reflection of parity itself but rather a reflection of other maternal factors that influence which women have more births. Therefore, when we examine typical j-shaped curves, which show the relationship between parity and pregnancy outcomes in a cross-sectional fashion (at a given point in time), it is important to consider the cohort of women contributing to each parity grouping.

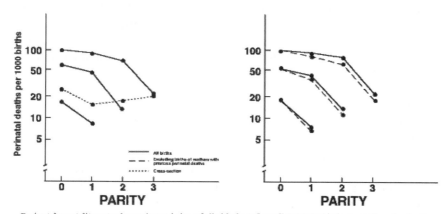

Perinatal mortality rates by parity and size of sibship based on all 137,919 births to mothers having two, three, or four singleton deliveries in Norway during the ten-year study period, 1967- 1976.(Left) Longitudinal and cross-sectional analyses of the data. (Right) Total longitudinal analysis compared to the longitudinal analysis after sibships containing previous perinatal deaths were excluded.

In the figure on the preceding page, the cross-sectional curve (dotted line in the first grid) suggests that the highest risk of perinatal mortality occurs among women of both low and high parity. When we examine the different cohorts of women contributing to this cross-sectional curve, however, we can see that the highest risk of perinatal mortality occurs at each birth among the cohort of women who are high parity when they complete their childbearing. For example, even the first infants born to these high parity women have an elevated mortality risk compared to the first infants born to women who remain at low parity. Also of interest is that within the high parity cohort, although each infant is at higher risk than infants in lower parity cohorts, the risk of perinatal death actually decreases with each subsequent birth. This relationship holds even when women with previous perinatal deaths are excluded from the analysis (second grid).

Place Characteristics

Place is central to epidemiology, whether the place demarcation is characterized using geo-political subdivisions or natural boundaries. When describing health events by geography, for example rates by county or proportions in urban versus rural areas, it is important to ascertain whether geographic differences represent unique features of the physical, social, economic, political, or health services environment. Public health professionals typically use geographic demarcations to compare how particular geo-political entities are faring with respect to health outcomes of interest. In addition, it is often necessary to identify if a health event or health outcome is clustered in a particular space, or in space and time. Usually, the objective is to identify whether the cluster reflects a true difference in exposure or a reflection of variations in population characteristics, variations in diagnosis and reporting, or variations in access to, utilization of, or effectiveness of health care services.

When using geographic characteristics to describe health events there are some issues that need to be considered.

Size and Level
When examining differences across geographical entities consideration should be given to the size and level of the political subdivisions to be compared. It is important to ascertain the level at which the relationship between a risk factor and an outcome is most salient as well as most amenable to intervention and to understand the different types of interventions possible at the various geographic levels such as county, city, or community area.

Availability and Stability of Data
When examining data in small geographic entities, either those that are physically large but have low population density, or those that are small by definition such as neighborhoods, it is essential to consider issues of data availability and data stability. In these situations it will probably be necessary to use techniques developed for small area analysis.

Time Characteristics

Examining trends over time is one of the most basic tools of epidemiology. It is a general assumption of Western culture that as our knowledge base and our technological skills grow over time, there should be a concomitant improvement in health outcomes. There is also the recognition that as new hazards emerge or as familiar hazards reach new populations, some health indicators may regress or deteriorate over time. As health professionals we are interested in exploring whether population characteristics, access to resources and health services, as well as health outcomes change over time. Of specific interest are changes in patterns of health events over long periods of time known as *secular trends*. Also of specific interest are patterns of health events that occur cyclically, such as seasonal occurrences. The greater incidence of SIDS (Sudden Infant Death Syndrome) in the late fall/early winter months is an example of a cyclically occurring health event.

When using time characteristics to describe health events there are some issues that need to be considered.

The Relationship Between Age and Time

When the overall rate of a health outcome is changing over time, care must be taken not to spuriously report a change in age-specific risks using cross-sectional data—data that includes many birth cohorts combined. The pattern of change in a health outcome is usually more accurately assessed using age-specific data for each birth cohort separately. This shift in analytic perspective is similar to that described earlier for examining the association between parity and perinatal outcome.

Members of a particular birth cohort may or may not experience historical phenomena or events such as the widespread availability of contraception or the emergence of HIV/AIDS, or they may experience these phenomena or events at very different points in the life cycle. When individuals from many birth cohorts are analyzed jointly, these varying experiences are masked. These varying experiences, however, are probably more important to understanding changes in age-specific risks over time than chronological age itself.

For example, during the 1960's and early 1970's, the incidence rate of endometrial cancer rose dramatically, particularly among women ages 45-64. This was not, however, a function of their age per se, but was due instead to the common experience of the cohort of women in this age group at that particular time in history. Many women in this cohort had been prescribed unopposed estrogens as a treatment for the symptoms of menopause. In late 1975, however, two papers documented the association between unopposed estrogens and endometrial cancer, and subsequently use of this treatment was sharply curtailed leading to a corresponding decrease in the rates of endometrial cancer in this age group.

Unopposed estrogen therapy had not been offered to women prior to the 1960's and early 1970's, and once estrogen therapy was identified as conferring cancer risk, it was of course not offered to women after 1975. If we looked at all women at one point in time, for example 1970, it might appear that women ages 45-64 were at increased risk for endometrial cancer; if, however, we looked separately at the different birth cohorts of women, we would see that this apparent increase in risk was an artifact.

As we've just seen, the time variable in epidemiology often reflects the effects of history. These effects include changes in culture, in the economy, in the political climate, in the use of technology, and advances in science as well as major historical events or interventions. For example, the introduction of surfactant in the very late 1980's is associated with the increased survival of very low birthweight infants. The forces of history as manifested by changes over time may have an independent association with health outcomes or may affect the manifestation of many individual risk factors or risk markers used to describe or explain health outcomes.

Question:

Think about an outcome of interest in your health agency. Can you describe the occurrence of this health outcome according to person, place, time?

Answer:

Example: Ectopic pregnancy

Ectopic pregnancy is defined as pregnancy occurring outside of the uterus, the most common type of which is tubal pregnancy. Ectopic pregnancy is the leading cause of maternal mortality in the first trimester of pregnancy, with case-fatality rates highest among young African-Americans. The following describes the occurrence of ectopic pregnancy according to person, place and time characteristics.

Person: rates are higher in older women, black women, women of low gravidity and parity.

Place: for the period 1970-1989, the highest rates of ectopic pregnancy were in the southern part of the US.

Time: there have been rising rates of ectopic pregnancy since the 1970's; this is a worldwide phenomenon.

STATISTICS USED IN PUBLIC HEALTH

Person, place and time variables are the building blocks used to describe and explain health events. These health events are summarized by public health statistics.

Types of Variables

Person, place, and time variables, as well as the health outcomes they describe, can take different forms. Variables with an infinite number of possible values (or so many it is difficult to list them) and whose values are ordered are said to be *continuous*. Variables with only a few possible values are said to be *discrete*. Sometimes discrete variables are derived from continuous ones by collapsing the many values into a few categories. Sometimes discrete variables are inherently discrete, having only two, three, or perhaps four possible values.

In practice, variables with a fairly limited number of possible values can be considered continuous as long as their values are ordered. Variables such as the number of well child visits in the first two years of life or the number of prenatal care visits fit this definition since the count of visits can be ranked. On the other hand, a variable such as county of residence has many possible values, but it cannot be considered continuous since the values have no intrinsic order or rank.

Variables such as well child visits or prenatal care visits are often transformed into discrete variables by defining categories such as < 5 visits, 5-9 visits, and >= 10 visits. Categories such as these are useful when it is believed that they capture distinct clinical, developmental, or programmatic groupings. While these values are still ordered, the natural ranking has been disrupted by the imposition of breakpoints and usually the variables derived in this fashion are considered discrete. Sometimes, in addition to capturing distinct groupings, variables are categorized because the ordering of the values is not applicable to a particular health issue being addressed. For instance, maternal age is chronologically ordered, yet this ordering is unsuitable for describing patterns of perinatal outcomes. Ages at both extremes of the reproductive age spectrum are associated with increased risk and therefore, maternal age is typically categorized into discrete groupings.

Other variables such as whether a child has a primary care provider, whether an infant is born with a congenital anomaly, whether a child dies, marital status, or county of residence are inherently discrete without any transformation. No ordering of any kind exists and breakpoints are imposed by the structure of the variables themselves.

Question:

Are the following variables discrete or continuous?

1. Type of practitioner seen for prenatal care e.g., obstetrician, family practitioner, or nurse/midwife
2. Apgar Scores
3. Number of days absent from school due to illness
4. Use of a bicycle helmet (yes or no)

Answer:

1. Discrete - no ordering
2. Continuous - limited number of values, but ordered
3. Continuous
4. Discrete - dichotomous

Means and Proportions

Statistics summarize information from continuous and discrete variables. The statistics used in maternal and child health are those used in other fields as well, most commonly means and proportions.

A *mean* is the sum of all observed values divided by the count of the total number of observations.

A *proportion* is the count of observations with a given value or set of values divided by the count of the total number of observations. Any observation counted in the numerator must also be counted in the denominator.

Means are used to summarize information from continuous variables; proportions are used to summarize information from discrete variables.

Suppose we have the following values from a small sample of 20 children for the number of well child visits in the first two years of life. We want to know the mean number of visits and we also want to know the proportion of children receiving fewer than five visits over the two-year period:

Variable **# Visits**				**Statistic: Mean # Visits** **Sum of Values / # Observations**	**Statistic: Proportion < 5 Visits** **Count of < 5 / # Observations**			
8	2	5	11	$8 + 2 + 5 + 11 + 6 + 0 + 4 + 5 +$	8	✓2	5	11
6	0	4	5	$7 + 14 + 7 + 8 + 8 + 1 + 4 + 6 +$	6	✓0	✓4	5
7	14	7	8	$\dfrac{10 + 9 + 6 + 3}{20}$	7	14	7	8
8	1	4	6		8	✓1	✓4	6
10	9	6	3	$= 6.2$	10	9	6	✓3

$$= \frac{6}{20} = 0.30$$

When a proportion is calculated from a variable such as well child visits, the original values are transformed into a discrete variable. The values to be counted in the numerator are either implicitly or explicitly assigned a new value of "1" and those with values not to be included in the numerator are assigned a new value of "0". When a variable is dichotomous with values of 1 and 0, summing and counting become equivalent and calculating the proportion is the same as calculating the mean. The values for a dichotomous variable for children receiving fewer than five visits are listed below along with the calculation of the mean/proportion:

Variable **< 5 Visits, Yes or No**				**Statistic: Mean/Proportion** **Sum or Count of Values / # of Observations**
0	1	0	0	$0 + 1 + 0 + 0 + 0 + 1 + 1 + 0 +$
0	1	1	0	$0 + 0 + 0 + 0 + 0 + 1 + 1 + 0 +$
0	0	0	0	$\dfrac{0 + 0 + 0 + 1}{20}$
0	1	1	0	
0	0	0	1	

$$\text{Mean/Prop.} = \frac{6}{20} = 0.30$$

Sometimes a series of proportions based on one variable is of interest. For instance, we may be interested in the proportion of children with fewer than five well child visits, the proportion of those with 5-9 visits, and the proportion with 10 or more visits. Again, a transformation or recoding of the original variable is necessary. There are several ways to do this:

Original Variable # Well Child Visits				Transformed into One Variable with 3 Values: < 5 visits =1 5-9 visits =2 10+ visits =3				Transformed into Two Dichotomous Variables: < 5 visits = 1,0 5-9 visits = 0,1 10 + visits = 0,0								
								< 5 Visits				5-9 Visits				10+ Visits	
8	2	5	11	2	1	2	3	0	1	0	0	1	0	1	0		
6	0	4	5	2	1	1	2	0	1	1	0	1	0	0	1	No need to
7	14	7	8	2	3	2	2	0	0	0	0	1	0	1	1	calculate
8	1	4	6	2	1	1	2	0	1	1	0	1	0	0	1	
10	9	6	3	3	2	2	1	0	0	0	1	0	1	1	0	

$$\frac{6}{20} = 0.30 \qquad \frac{11}{20} = 0.55 \qquad \frac{3}{20} = 0.15$$

If well child visits is recoded into one variable with the values of 1, 2, and 3, proportions must be calculated by *counting* how many times a "1" occurs, how many times a "2" occurs, and how many times a "3" occurs. If, instead, the recoding is accomplished by creating two dichotomous variables, then *summing* and *counting* are once again equivalent.

While three proportions are of interest here, only two dichotomous variables are needed to capture the information we want. The dichotomous coding allows us to sum the number of children coded "1" on the first variable and sum the number coded "1" on the second variable in order to calculate the proportion of children with fewer than 5 visits and the number with 5-9 visits. Once we know that these proportions equal 0.30 and 0.55, we automatically know that the proportion of children with 10 or more visits equals 0.15 since, by definition, each proportion lies between 0.00 and 1.00, and their total exactly equals 1.00. The last proportion can also be arrived at by counting the number of children coded "0" on both variables.

────Comment

Notice that with a sample size of 20, it is only feasible to construct an example for a fairly large proportion such as 0.30. For rare events, a large sample or population is required before a proportion can be reported. With a sample size of 20, examining any proportion less than 0.05 (1 / 20) will be meaningless because, on average, no event will be observed. For example, the probability of observing a child fatality due to injury in a sample size of 20 is close to 0.

Question:

What is the mean length of stay, in hours, following delivery for the following sample of 20 women?

64	32	54	21
23	40	17	45
55	20	48	67
48	86	46	19
84	109	95	51

Answer:

51.2 hours

Question:

What is the proportion of women whose hospital stay was < 24 hours?

Answer:

5 / 20 = 0.25 or 25 %

Question:

Recode length of stay into 2 dichotomous variables (values of 1 and 0) that describe the proportions of women whose stays were < 24 hours, 24 to < 48 hours, and >=48 hours.

Answer:

< 24 hours					24 to < 48 hours			
0	0	0	1		0	1	0	0
1	0	1	0		0	1	0	1
0	1	0	0		0	0	0	0
0	0	0	1		0	0	1	0
0	0	0	0		0	0	0	0

25%	< 24 hours
20%	24 to < 48 hours
55%	>= 48 hours

Rates

Of particular interest in public health is a special class of statistics called rates. In mathematical terms, a *rate* is a proportion in which the denominator is not a count of individuals, but rather a sum of the varying amounts of time each individual was observed. The denominator, therefore, is expressed in person-time units such as person hours, person days, or person years. This definition of a rate is typically relaxed to include proportions with counts of individuals in the denominator linked to a certain time period, for example the total number of live births in a year. In this case, each infant, regardless of how long it survives, is considered to be observed for the entire year.

Like any proportion, observations counted in the numerator of a rate must also be counted or their observation time summed in the denominator. Unlike some proportions, however, all of the observations included in the denominator of a rate must also have the potential for being counted in the numerator. In epidemiologic terms, all of the observations included in the denominator of a rate must be *at risk* for being included in the numerator.

Ratios, Proportions, and Rates

A *ratio* is any division of one number by another; the numerator and denominator do not have to be mutually exclusive.

A *proportion* is a ratio in which those in the numerator are also in the denominator.

A *rate* is a ratio in which those in the numerator are also in the denominator, and those in the denominator are "at risk" of being in the numerator. The denominator is the sum of "at risk" person-time or, by convention, the count of individuals "at risk" in a given time period.

Sometimes, indicators that do not meet even the relaxed definition of a rate are nonetheless called rates by convention. Following is a brief discussion of two such indicators commonly used in MCH—the infant mortality rate and the postneonatal mortality rate.

When an infant mortality rate is calculated using the infant deaths during a calendar year together with the live births in the same calendar year (period method), the resulting "rate" does not conform to the definition of a proportion nor to that for a rate. Since some infants born in one calendar year die in the following one, infants counted in the numerator and denominator are different infants and following from this, all infants in the denominator are not at risk for being counted in the numerator. An infant mortality rate that at least meets the relaxed definition of a rate, on the other hand, is calculated using data for a unique birth cohort—linking individual infant death certificates to the matching birth certificates (cohort method).

The standard calculation of a postneonatal mortality rate likewise results in a measure that technically is not a "rate". Typically, all live births are included in the denominator of a postneonatal mortality rate despite the fact that infants who die during the neonatal period are not at risk of dying during the postneonatal period.

Some MCH epidemiologists are recommending reporting postneonatal mortality excluding the neonatal deaths from the denominator. If this recommendation were implemented, the smaller denominator would result in higher reported postneonatal mortality.

$$\frac{\text{\# postneonatal deaths}}{\text{\# live births - \# neonatal deaths}} > \frac{\text{\# postneonatal deaths}}{\text{\# live births}}$$

On the other hand, using the "incorrect" definition of postneonatal mortality has some advantages. With all live births as a common denominator for neonatal, postneonatal and infant mortality, it is possible to report proportionate mortality:

Proportion of Infant Mortality Occurring in the Postneonatal Period

$$\frac{\text{Postneonatal Mortality Rate}}{\text{Infant Mortality Rate}} = \frac{\dfrac{\text{\# postneonatal deaths}}{\text{\# live births}}}{\dfrac{\text{\# infant deaths}}{\text{\# live births}}} = \frac{\text{\# postneonatal deaths}}{\text{\# infant deaths}}$$

This calculation could not be done if the denominators in the rates were different.

Throughout thi   xt, we will use a relaxed definition of the term rate, noting the implications of doing so as well. Clarity in defining numerators and denominators is an essential step in developing meaningful MCH indicators of health status, health services, and health systems.

Question:

Decide which of the following are *rates*, giving reasons for why they do or do not meet the appropriate criteria.

1. the number of births to adolescents as a proportion of all live births
2. the proportion of two-year-old children who have had < 5 well child visits during a year.
3. the number of pediatric beds as a proportion of total hospital beds

Answer:

1. This is not a rate, since the majority of live births counted in the denominator are to women who are not adolescents. A rate of adolescent childbearing will have only adolescents in the denominator.
2. This is a rate, since all two-year-olds are at risk for having minimal visits and time is part of the measure.
3. This is not a rate since beds are fixed items, not events occurring in time.

Question:

What is the appropriate denominator if hospitalizations for injury among children are in the numerator?

Answer:

Different denominators might be appropriate depending on the issue being addressed. The total number of children in the population might be used as the denominator to yield a population rate of hospitalization for injury. On the other hand, the denominator might include only those children who have had an injury to yield a rate of childhood injury that highlights the extent of injuries severe enough to require hospitalization. As this example illustrates, definition of the population at risk is not always clear cut.

Prevalence and Incidence

The discussion of proportions and rates is further refined by the epidemiologic concepts of prevalence and incidence. Considerations surrounding how disease and death occur in populations have led to some specialized measures of occurrence.

In our everyday public health discourse, we continually report rates that describe the extent of a phenomenon in a community, or that describe the impact of a health event on a community. While we don't often take the time to label these rates as such, we are usually reporting prevalence rates or incidence rates. While similar in outward appearance, prevalence and incidence rates tell different stories, and therefore it is important to distinguish between them.

Prevalence Rates

Prevalence rates estimate the proportion of individuals in a population who have the outcome or have experienced the event of interest at a specific point in time.

Prevalence rates are typically derived from cross-sectional surveys and as such are concerned with existing cases of a health outcome at a point in time; they provide an estimate of the probability of having a health status outcome or event at a given time. Because these rates describe the burden of illness in a population, public health professionals use prevalence rates to gather information about the impact of a health event on the resource needs of the health care delivery system. The number of cases of childhood asthma in the total population of children in a given year, or the number of cases of adolescent substance use in the total population of adolescents in a given year are examples of prevalence rates.

Prevalence Rate

$$= \frac{\text{\# of individuals with a health condition}}{\text{\# of individuals in the relevant population}} \text{ at a given point in time}$$

Example : Asthma Prevalence in Children < 18

$$= \frac{\text{\# of children} < 18 \text{ with asthma}}{\text{\# of children} < 18} \text{ as reported in annual survey}$$

Incidence Rates

Incidence rates quantify the number of new events or cases of an outcome that develop in a population of individuals at risk for that outcome during a specified time interval. They also provide a direct measure of the rate at which new illness occurs in the population and as such incidence rates and the incident cases from which they are derived can be used to study the etiology of health events. For instance, to study the relationship between the introduction of a toxic waste dump into a community and the development of asthma in children, it would be necessary to either retrospectively or prospectively gather incident cases of asthma. In other words, data would be collected on children who were free from asthma at the beginning of the time period of interest, i.e., before the toxic waste dump began operation.

There are two measures of incidence that are commonly used, cumulative incidence and incidence density.

Cumulative Incidence. The number of new cases of a health outcome or event during a given period of time among the population at risk is called *cumulative incidence*. Cumulative incidence rates provide an estimate of the probability or risk that an individual will develop an outcome or experience an event during a specified time period. If the population not at risk is also included in the denominator one is likely to underestimate the risk of the event or outcome. For example, if a local school system is interested in correctly documenting the risk of primary grade children developing vision problems during a given school year, students who are already diagnosed with vision problems would be excluded from both the numerator and denominator.

Cumulative Incidence Rate

$$= \frac{\text{\# of new cases of a health outcome during a given period of time}}{\text{\# at risk of developing the outcome at the start of the period}}$$

Example: Cumulative Incidence of Asthma in Children < 18

$$= \frac{\text{\# of new cases of asthma in children} < 18 \text{ during a year}}{\text{\# of children} < 18 \text{ without asthma at the start of the year}}$$

Incidence Density. The number of new cases of an event or an outcome that occur during a given period of time in relation to the total person-time of observation is known as *incidence density*. Incidence density is a rate in the strictest definition of this term because it accounts for the amount of time each individual in the population at risk is actually observed. Each individual contributes to the denominator only for the amount of time they are disease free. This measure is also called the *force of morbidity* or *mortality* because it provides an estimate of the instantaneous rate of development of the outcome in the population.

Incidence Density

$$= \frac{\text{\# new cases of a health outcome}}{\text{Total person time of observation}} \text{ during a given period of time}$$

Example: Asthma Incidence Density in Children < 18

$$= \frac{\text{\# new cases of asthma in children} < 18 \text{ during the year}}{\text{Sum of the asthma - free time during the year for each child}}$$

Because cumulative incidence approximates incidence density when the true or underlying incidence is low (i.e., the force of morbidity or mortality is not great) or the time period of observation is short, health professionals most often use cumulative incidence rates because they are more easily calculated. For example, we've seen that an infant mortality rate could theoretically be calculated so that the denominator is the sum of the survival time each infant contributes. However, because infant death is a relatively rare event, using this more complicated denominator instead of simply the count of the total number of infants will not yield a substantially different measure than the cumulative incidence rate.

In fact, very few public health professionals have the luxury of measuring the time each individual contributes to a cohort's experience. Rather we have information about the total number of births or the total population in a geographic area during a given year so that person-time measures are rarely reported in standard public health surveillance. Incidence density rates seem to be most useful when there is rapid accumulation of cases such as in an infectious disease outbreak.

Prevalence and incidence are related in the following way:

$$\text{Prevalence} \cong \text{Incidence} \times \text{Duration}$$

Because prevalence depends on both incidence and the duration of the health outcome or event in the population, high prevalence does not imply an increased risk of the outcome of interest but rather may indicate long duration or improved survival. Similarly, low prevalence is not equivalent to low incidence but rather may represent a rapid fatal process or a rapid cure. It should also be noted that mortality rates are a special case in which there really is no difference between incidence and prevalence, since death can only occur once and has no duration, so that the above formula becomes:

$$\text{Prevalence} = \text{Incidence} \times 0$$
or
$$\text{Prevalence} = \text{Incidence}$$

In practice, mortality rates are considered incidence rates.

Comment

If we want to calculate the infant mortality rate according to the strictest definition (as incidence density), those infants who survive the entire year of interest will contribute one full year to the denominator, while those infants who die during the year of interest will contribute only the portion of the year for which they were alive. Since the denominator of this rate will be somewhat smaller than that commonly reported, the resulting infant mortality rate will be somewhat higher.

$$\frac{\#\,\text{infant deaths}}{\text{Sum of "infant years" observed}} > \frac{\#\,\text{infant deaths}}{\#\,\text{live births}}$$

Question:

All of the following are rates. Determine whether each is a cumulative incidence or a prevalence rate.

1. Age-specific asthma mortality rate
2. Rate of smoking among adolescents
3. Infant mortality rate
4. Proportion of women who are newly uninsured
5. Age-specific asthma morbidity rate
6. Proportion of children who are uninsured
7. Rates of vaccine preventable diseases
8. Proportion of children who have activity limitations

Answer:

	Reason
1. cumulative incidence	A mortality rate is an incidence rate
2. prevalence	Counts all current cases
3. cumulative incidence	A mortality rate is an incidence rate
4. cumulative incidence	Counts only new cases
5. prevalence	Counts all current cases
6. prevalence	Counts all current cases
7. cumulative incidence	Counts only new cases
8. prevalence	Counts all current cases

CHOOSING STATISTICS TO REPORT

In public health, proportions and rates are often more useful statistics to report than are means. Birthweight is a clear example of a variable that is close to being truly continuous, yet is routinely transformed into a discrete variable for reporting purposes. Infants are typically classified into categories of < 1500 grams, 1500-2499 grams, and >= 2500 grams under the assumption that these breakpoints delineate groups with homogeneous health status. Because the vast majority of infants are born >= 2500 grams, reporting mean birthweight will not reveal much about the extent of high risk births, whereas reporting the rate of low birthweight or that of very low birthweight separates out the high risk births and brings them into sharper focus.

For example, the mean birthweight among all births in one year might be 3,200 grams. This statistic, however, tells us little about the extent of low birthweight. In fact, two populations, one with a low birthweight rate of 6 % and one with a low birthweight rate of 12 % might have mean birthweights of 3,300 and 3,100 grams respectively. Showing that the presence of a risk factor lowers mean birthweight by an average of 200 grams across the entire birthweight distribution is a far less forceful statement than showing that the presence of a risk factor doubles the likelihood of an infant being < 2,500 grams. Using birthweight in its continuous form, then, could hinder development of appropriately targeted public health interventions.

From a statistical perspective, when continuous variables are transformed into discrete ones, there is loss of information. If children who had fewer than five well child visits are combined into one category, we lose the ability to explore differences between children who, for example, had zero visits and those who had four visits. When infants born at 700 grams are combined with those born at 2,000 grams, we lose the ability to explore differences between them. This loss of information is counteracted, however, if there is a substantial gain in public health meaning.

Comment and Example

Choosing statistics to report may also depend on the type of data-set available for analysis. Observations in a public health data-set may be individual women, infants or children, or they may be households, clinics, neighborhoods, counties, the state or the nation. That is, a data-set may contain records with values for individuals, or it may contain records with group statistics, aggregated according to some criterion such as residence in an area, enrollment in a health plan, or classification into a demographic category.

All statistics can be thought of as weighted averages; an unweighted average simply means that the weights are all equal. When individual level data are being analyzed, each individual is given equal weight in the calculation of statistics. When aggregate level data are being analyzed, each group, such as a county, can either be considered an "individual" and given equal weight in the calculation of statistics, or it can be differentially weighted according to the number of actual individuals represented within it.

If equal weight is given to each group, then the summary means or proportions that are computed are statistics that summarize other statistics—for instance, the mean of a series of county means, the mean of a series of county proportions, the mean of a series of county rates, or the proportion of a series of county proportions above or below a certain cutpoint.

In contrast, if each group is weighted according to the number of individuals within it, then the summary means or proportions that are computed are the same as those that would have been computed had individual level data been available. In order to do this using an aggregate level data-set, the counts of individuals in the numerators and denominators must be available as well as the corresponding group means, proportions, or rates.

For example, using county level data from a state, the mean of the series of county child injury fatality rates might be of interest, or the overall state child injury fatality rate might be of interest. These two statistics—an unweighted rate and a rate weighted by the child population in each county—are often quite different and may tell a different story.

Returning to the data on the number of well child visits for 20 hypothetical children used previously to illustrate the calculation of means and proportions, recall that the mean number of visits was found to be 6.2. Because these data were for individuals, each child's value was given the same "weight" of 1/20 (or 0.05) and the unweighted mean could be written as:

$$\frac{1}{20}8 + \frac{1}{20}2 + \frac{1}{20}5 + \frac{1}{20}11 + \frac{1}{20}6 + \frac{1}{20}0 + \frac{1}{20}4 + \frac{1}{20}5 + \frac{1}{20}7 + \frac{1}{20}14 +$$

$$\frac{1}{20}7 + \frac{1}{20}8 + \frac{1}{20}8 + \frac{1}{20}1 + \frac{1}{20}4 + \frac{1}{20}6 + \frac{1}{20}10 + \frac{1}{20}9 + \frac{1}{20}6 + \frac{1}{20}3$$

$$= \frac{8 + 2 + 5 + 11 + 6 + 0 + 4 + 5 + 7 + 14 + 7 + 8 + 8 + 1 + 4 + 6 + 10 + 9 + 6 + 3}{20}$$

$$= 6.2$$

Now suppose we want to know the mean number of well child visits among two-year-olds in a health region with 20 counties. Assume that the same 20 values seen before for the 20 individuals are now the mean number of well child visits in each of 20 counties. Below are the hypothetical county level data:

1. County	2. Population of Children Age 2	3. Total Number of Well Child Visits	4. Mean # Well Child Visits	5. Proportion of Total Population of Children Age 2 in Each County (Weights)
1	65,000	520,000	8	0.039
2	13,000	26,000	2	0.008
3	8,500	42,500	5	0.005
4	285,000	3,135,000	11	0.172
5	2,500	15,000	6	0.002
6	1,250	0	0	0.001
7	6,000	24,000	4	0.004
8	3,750	18,750	5	0.002
9	10,500	73,500	7	0.006
10	375,000	5,250,000	14	0.226
11	125,000	875,000	7	0.075
12	75,000	600,000	8	0.045
13	87,500	700,000	8	0.053
14	4,500	4,500	1	0.003
15	3,800	15,200	4	0.002
16	5,750	34,500	6	0.003
17	250,000	2,500,000	10	0.151
18	225,000	2,025,000	9	0.136
19	100,000	600,000	6	0.060
20	9,500	28,500	3	0.006
Total	**1,656,550**	**16,487,450**	**124**	**1.000**

The mean number of well child visits in each county is the total number of well child visits in each county divided by the total population of children age 2 in each county (column 3 / column 2). The weight for each county is the total population of children age 2 in each county divided by the total for all 20 counties combined (column 2 / total of column 2).

With these aggregate data, both an unweighted or a weighted mean can be calculated. If each county is considered an individual, then the unweighted mean will again be 6.2 calculated in exactly the same way as it was for the individual children. The sample size is again 20, and the weights are again all 0.05.

To account for the different numbers of two-year-olds in the 20 counties, an overall or weighted mean can be calculated using the sample size of 1,656,550 two-year-olds in all 20 counties, and the 16,487,450 total well child visits as follows:

$$\text{Weighted Mean} = \frac{16,487,450}{1,656,550} = 9.95$$

This calculation can be rewritten to explicitly show the incorporation of the weights corresponding to each county's proportionate share of the population of 2-year-olds:

$$(0.039\times8)+(0.008\times2)+(0.005\times5)+(0.172\times11)+(0.002\times6)+(0.001\times0)+$$

$$(0.004\times4)+(0.002\times5)+(0.006\times7)+(0.226\times14)+(0.075\times7)+(0.045\times8)+$$

$$(0.053\times8)+(0.003\times1)+(0.002\times4)+(0.003\times6)+(0.151\times10)+(0.136\times9)+$$

$$(0.060\times6)+(0.006\times3)$$

$$=\frac{16,487,450}{1,656,550}$$

$$=9.95$$

The difference between the weighted mean of 9.95 and the unweighted mean of 6.2 reflects the differential health care experience of the children in the 20 counties; children in counties with larger populations tended to receive a greater number of well child visits than those in counties with smaller populations. Which mean best describes the experience in the 20 counties combined? The answer depends on the question being asked. If the question is, "On average, how many well child visits has each two-year-old in the region received?" then the weighted or overall mean, which is based on individuals, is most appropriate. If, however, the question is, "On average, how many well child visits have county health care systems delivered to children by the age of 2?" then the unweighted mean may be appropriate.

Defining Categories

The goal when categorizing variables is to identify breakpoints that make sense clinically and programmatically so that services and policies can be aimed at the average experience reflected in the chosen groupings. The more homogenous the groupings the better, because then the average information these contain is more likely to be a reasonable reflection of the underlying continuous data they summarize. The impact of the loss of information, then, will be minimized.

Below are examples of person, place, and time variables illustrating the different forms each might take, ranging from almost continuous to simply dichotomous:

Person (maternal age)	Place	Time
10,11,12,13…42,43,44,45 …	Individual Addresses	Days
10-14,15-17,18-19,20-24, 25-29,30-34,35-39,40-44,45 +	Blocks	Weeks
10-14,15-17,18-19,20-29, 30-34,35-39,40 +	Block Groups	Months
10-14,15-19,20-29,30-39,40 +	Census Tracts	Years
< 20,20-29,30-39,40 +	Counties	Two Year Groups
< 20,20-34,35 +	Groups of Counties	Five Year Groups
< 20 v. >= 20	Urban v. Rural	Pre 1989 v. Post 1989

There are several approaches to choosing categories, including using the observed distribution of the values or using a conceptual or clinical framework. Each of these involves a counting strategy that assigns a value into a given category. Sometimes, the desired breakpoints are generated automatically out of computer software as descriptive statistics such as quartiles or the median, or sometimes computer programming statements are necessary to achieve appropriate assignments. When sample size is small, assignments may be calculated by hand.

Using the Observed Distribution of the Data

Often, the categories generated are based on the distribution of the observed data. The figure below shows four ways that values of a variable might be distributed. Let's assume that the 20 values are rates ranging from 0 to 100 for 20 counties. Quartiles are marked in each case, breaking the 20 data points into four categories with five observations in each.

Quartiles of Four Possible Distributions
Values (+) for 20 Hypothetical Counties

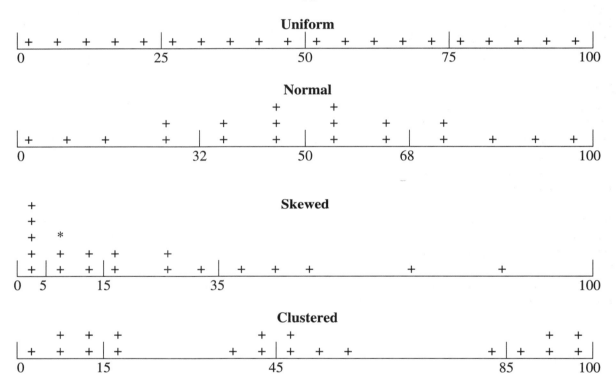

Following are three ways to create categories using the observed distribution in the data:

Equal Counts. If the data are close to uniformly distributed (there are equivalent numbers of data points along the entire range of values), then it may be reasonable to use quartiles, quintiles, or other percentiles that divide the observed data into groups with equal sample size.

Looking at the figure above, you can see that for uniformly distributed data these quartile groupings may make sense, but that particularly when data are skewed (very unevenly distributed) or when data are clustered, using quartiles results in some categories being very narrow, containing only very similar rates, and other categories being very wide, containing very different rates. For instance, in the skewed distribution, the counties with rates of approximately 3 and 7 are grouped separately in the first and second categories, while counties with rates all the way from 35-100 are grouped together in the fourth category.

Equal Ranges. To insure homogeneous groupings, sometimes breakpoints are based on ranges of the observed data. Rather than obtaining equal numbers of observations in each category, this approach results in equal portions of the range in each category. If four categories are desired, for example, then the range is divided into four equal parts. For uniformly distributed values, there is no difference between obtaining equal counts or equal ranges, but for a skewed distribution, the categories defined by the range will be very different than those defined by counts. For the skewed distribution in the above figure, if categories are defined according to the range of rates to include counties with rates of 0-24, 25-49, 50-74, and 75-100, then the first category would contain 12 of the 20 counties and the fourth category would contain only one. These groupings may be a better representation of meaningful differences in health risks and outcomes.

Naturally Occurring Breakpoints. Looking closely at the distribution of observed values may reveal that neither equal numbers of observations nor equal portions of the range will yield homogeneous categories. The data might be clustered so that naturally occurring breaks are evident. In the example of clustered data in the figure above, using this approach would mean defining only three categories, with breakpoints at approximately 35 and 65.

Using Conceptual Breakpoints

Categories may also be defined according to conceptual breakpoints corresponding to clinical, economic, social or cultural standards regardless of the observed distribution in the data. As seen in the following table, the commonly used categories for birthweight discussed earlier do not contain equal numbers of infants, nor equal portions of the range of possible birthweights, nor even natural clustering of birthweights typically observed in vital records data. They do, however, reflect a clinical interpretation of the data that addresses public health concerns.

Similarly, initiation of prenatal care is often categorized by trimester because the effectiveness of this set of services is believed to be enhanced when women access care early in pregnancy. The table below illustrates that this categorization of prenatal care utilization is not a reflection of the distribution of the observed data. Fully 85% of the women begin care in the first trimester and are grouped together, rather than a maximum of 25% that would be imposed by using quartiles. Instead, the categories are a reflection of programmatic characteristics.

Approximate Percent Distributions of Observed Values of Birthweight and Initiation of Prenatal Care Commonly Used Categories

Birthweight		Initiation of Prenatal Care	
< 1500 grams	2.0	1st Trimester	85.0
1500-2499	5.0	2nd Trimester	10.0
2500 +	93.0	3rd Trimester	3.0
		No Prenatal Care	2.0

Question:

Here are the sorted values for the parity of 20 women. How would you describe the distribution? Is it uniform, normal, skewed, clustered? If you wanted to categorize the values, how many categories would you choose and where would the breakpoints for those categories be?

0 0 0 0 1 1 1 1 1 1 2 2 2 2 3 3 4 4 6 8

Answer:

The distribution of the values is skewed, with most women at low parity and only a few with very high parity. In addition, differing parities carry different clinical and programmatic meaning. A possible categorization strategy would be to define 3 categories, separating out nulliparous women as well as women with very high parity. The categories could be 0, 1-4, and> 4.

THE SAMPLING FRAMEWORK

The methods used to analyze commonly used statistics such as means, proportions, and rates come from sampling theory, resting on the assumption that a random sample of observations has been drawn from an infinite population. This assumption defines a landscape in which exact measurement is never possible, a landscape in which statistics summarize information from only one of an infinite number of possible samples that could be selected from a population.

While the goal of sampling is to obtain a subset of observations with characteristics that mirror those in the whole population, this goal cannot be fully realized. Each sample that is drawn will be different from any other sample drawn, yielding slightly different statistics simply due to chance. For example, the mean age or the range in income levels or the total number of children with disabilities will vary from sample to sample since any given member of a population could be selected in one instance but not in another. Statistics, then, only approximate the true population values they represent.

Accounting for the uncertainty and inaccuracy—the sampling error—inherent in our data is at the heart of statistical analysis. Random sampling, in which each individual has an equal and independent chance of being selected from the population of interest, is a method that minimizes sampling error, but even with random sampling, error cannot be completely eliminated. Finding exact answers to our questions about the health and health care of women, infants, and children is not possible given this link between statistics and sampling. Instead, our task is to make reasonable *estimates* of the occurrence of health events and then to generate and test hypotheses about the relationships between these and other factors.

The assumptions and definitions from classical statistical theory are often confusing when applied to the analysis of public health data. For instance, all of the following are considered "populations" and not "samples" used for reporting health statistics:

- All residents of the U.S. in 1997
- All live births in a state in 1997
- All women ages 15-44 in a city in 1997
- All children ages 0-3 below 185% of the poverty level in a city in June-August 1997.

Accounting for sampling error in this context may seem unnecessary since no sample has been drawn, and in fact indicators generated from these populations are often presented in surveillance and other reports as being exact population values.

For example, an annual infant mortality rate in an area is based on the known number of infant deaths and the known total number of live births. No sample, random or otherwise, is drawn to generate this indicator. Similarly, the annual rate of pediatric hospital discharges in an area is based on the known number of discharges occurring to patients under age 21 and the known total census of children under 21 in the year of interest. Again, no sample is drawn to generate this indicator.

In actuality, though, we never have access to an entire population, even if that population is finite as in the examples above. Even the U.S. Census, for instance, falls short of complete coverage, and therefore values generated from these data can be considered sample statistics or estimates. In fact, it is thought that a formal sampling strategy for the Census would yield more accurate estimates of population characteristics than those resulting from attempted complete enumeration.

Moreover, finite populations such as all live births or all children under 21 can be thought of as samples in time and space. A live birth occurring in December of one year at 37 weeks gestation had a chance of occurring in January of the following year at 41 weeks gestation, becoming a member of a different population. Or a high-risk infant may survive or die depending on a host of factors known and unknown, thus changing the count of infant deaths. In addition, sampling from January through December to generate an annual infant mortality rate is itself arbitrary. Why not sample from July through June?

Similarly, a hospital discharge from a given institution had a chance of occurring in another location depending on a host of factors relating to diagnosis, medical decision-making, and service delivery issues. Or it may not have occurred at all. In addition, the population of children under 21 is likely to be continuously changing as a result of in-migration and out-migration. The reported hospitalization rate, therefore, is an estimate of the true rate within the context of a dynamic environment.

These examples illustrate that if history could be rerun, the number of infant deaths, live births, pediatric hospitalizations, and the child population might be different for a given place and time than what is reported from population data. This kind of error is usually called random error rather than sampling error since no sample is explicitly drawn, but regardless of the label, chance plays a role in what data we observe.

The extent of error in the estimates we report, whether these estimates are derived from sample data or population data, is related to the number of observations available to compute them. In large samples, error is likely to be small because each member of the population has a high probability of being included, and therefore it is likely the sample will have within it the complex combinations of characteristics contained in the population. In large populations, error is also likely to be small because the impact of random variability due to unknowable factors will be minimized. Conversely, the extent of error in small samples or small populations may be substantial due either to the increased likelihood that a given sample is unrepresentative or the increased impact of random variability.

As public health professionals focus on smaller geographic areas and smaller populations to better target interventions, addressing the potential for error in estimates of health risks and outcomes becomes a critical part of the decision-making process. If data are to be examined by census tract, for example, the numbers of health events will be quite small and the potential error quite large. Any programmatic strategy has to take this into account.

We recommend that analysis of all health data be anchored by the framework of sampling theory regardless of whether the data come from a sample or a population and regardless of the sample or population size. The process of evaluating and reporting the extent of error allows us to differentiate between "good" data and "bad" data and therefore base our decisions on strong rather than weak evidence. Acknowledging the uncertainty in all data helps to insure that the accuracy and meaning of health information is consciously addressed and challenged, rather than simply assumed.

Comment and Example

Suppose there is a population of 50 children under age 5 in a community who have been diagnosed with asthma, and assume that this number reflects complete case ascertainment. The column below displaying the "actual data" shows how many and which of these children were actually hospitalized during one year. A "1" indicates that hospitalization occurred. Since this is not a sample, it might be assumed that if the experience of these children in the given year could be observed multiple times with all known conditions remaining unchanged, the hospitalization pattern would be identical. However, the data below for this hypothetical situation shows that this may not be the case.

Child #	Actual Data 1.	Hypothetical Data if History Could be Rerun 2.	3.	4.
1	0	0	0	0
2	0	0	0	0
3	0	0	0	0
4	0	0	0	0
5	1	1	0	1
6	0	0	0	0
7	0	0	0	0
8	0	0	0	0
9	0	0	0	0
10	0	0	0	0
11	0	0	0	0
12	0	0	0	1
13	2	1	2	1
14	0	0	0	0
15	0	0	0	0
16	0	0	0	0
17	0	0	0	0
18	0	0	0	0
19	0	0	0	0
20	0	0	0	0
21	0	0	0	0
22	0	0	0	0
23	0	0	0	0
24	0	0	0	0
25	0	1	0	0
26	0	0	0	0
27	0	0	0	0
28	0	0	0	0
29	0	0	0	0
30	0	0	1	0
31	0	0	0	0
32	0	0	0	0
33	0	0	0	0
34	0	0	0	0
35	0	0	0	0
36	0	1	0	1
37	0	0	0	0
38	0	0	0	0
39	1	1	0	0
40	0	0	0	0
41	0	0	0	0
42	0	0	0	0
43	0	0	0	0
44	0	0	0	0
45	0	0	0	0
46	0	0	0	0
47	0	0	0	0
48	0	0	0	0
49	0	0	0	0
50	0	0	0	0
Total Hospitalizations	4	5	3	4
Hospitalization Rate	$\frac{4}{50} \times 100 = 8$	$\frac{5}{50} \times 100 = 10$	$\frac{3}{50} \times 100 = 6$	$\frac{4}{50} \times 100 = 8$

The asthma hospitalization rates seen in columns 1-3 are different—8, 10, and 6 per 100 respectively. In addition, although the rates in columns 1 and 4 are the same, the individual children who are hospitalized are different. There are always unknowable factors that make an indicator subject to a certain degree of variability. What might account for this variability? It might be that a physician's decision for child #36 in column 1 was that, though borderline, hospitalization was not warranted, whereas in column 2 the decision for the same child was the reverse. The parents' decision to see a doctor during an episode may also vary, and/or the level of environmental pollution may vary depending on the weather and other conditions. No sampling error exists in this example, since all children with asthma are known and followed. Instead, what is illustrated is "random error".

EVALUATING THE ACCURACY OF STATISTICS

Statistical theory identifies probability distributions that describe how the values of a statistic would change if different samples (an infinite number of them) were drawn from a population. These distributions provide a frame of reference for judging the accuracy of estimates.

A *probability distribution* (or relative frequency distribution) is based on a set of mathematical rules that define the likelihood that a value or set of values will actually be observed in a sample. When a variable is discrete, a probability can be determined for observing each possible value. When a variable is continuous, probabilities are determined for a range of values.

In order to evaluate the accuracy of the means and proportions we report we need to understand the probability distributions of these statistics. While we observe a distribution of values on each unique variable for the individuals in our sample, we do not observe a distribution of values for the means and proportions that summarize the data: we only see one instance of each statistic from our single sample. Instead, statistical theory specifies probability distributions that describe how statistics commonly used in public health are expected to vary across many potential samples. We know from theory that it is extremely unlikely that the one statistic we observe will exactly equal the true population value; by using the appropriate probability distribution we can assess how far our estimate may be from the actual experience in the population.

In the example of number of well child visits used previously, recall that the mean was calculated to be 6.2 visits based on 20 observations and the proportion of children with fewer than five visits was calculated to be 30 % from the same sample. Now we can refer to known probability distributions to describe theoretically how all of the possible means and proportions from samples of this size are expected to be distributed. We can then assess whether 6.2 visits is a reasonable summary of the amount of well child care children under age two are receiving, and whether 30 % is a reasonable summary of the extent of minimal utilization of care.

The following probability distributions describe how commonly used statistics are distributed:

- Normal
- Binomial
- Poisson
- Chi-square
- F
- Exponential

These distributions are related to each other—they are all members of what is called the exponential family. The similarity among three of the distributions can be seen in the shapes of the curves for the t, X^2, and F distributions.

t Distribution with 10 Degrees of Freedom (d.f.)

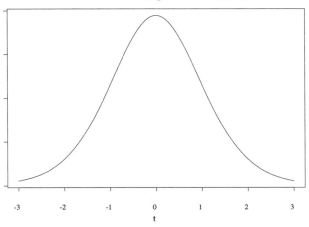

Chi-Square Distributions

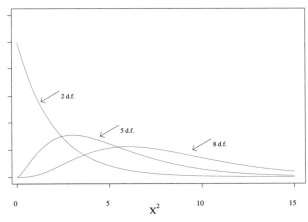

F Distributions
Denominator d.f. = 20

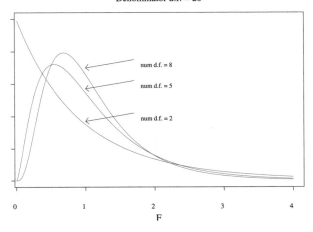

Means are generally assumed to follow a *normal distribution*. Proportions are assumed to follow the *Binomial distribution*. A proportion is also said to be *Poisson* distributed if its numerator is very small compared to its denominator. Many prevalence and incidence rates used as public health statistics fit this description. When rates are expressed per 1,000, 10,000, or 100,000 because of the low frequency of the health outcome they are measuring, they are treated as Poisson variables.

The Mean and Variance of Probability Distributions

The two defining characteristics or parameters of a probability distribution are its mean and variance. Together, these two measures determine the accuracy of a statistic. Remember that when the probability distribution is of a summary statistic, then the individual values on the distribution are the means, proportions, or rates from each of the infinite hypothetical samples. The *mean* of the distribution is the mean of these means, proportions or rates, and the *variance* is the variance of these means, proportions, or rates.

$$\text{Accuracy} = \text{Bias} + \text{Reliability}$$

Bias: Does the *mean* of the series of hypothetical estimates obtained from repeated sampling equal the true population value?

Reliability: Is the *variance* of the series of hypothetical estimates obtained from repeated sampling small enough so that the observed estimate is probably close to the true population value?

The statistical bias of an estimate can rarely be assessed directly. Instead, statistical theory is relied upon to show that commonly used statistics are unbiased. Sample means, proportions, and rates, for example, are theoretically unbiased estimates of true population values. In fact, we have come to use these statistics precisely because they are theoretically unbiased.

Means and Variances for Means, Proportions, and Rates

The following formulas show that the expected values of means, proportions, and rates are each the mean of a particular probability distribution. The expected value of a mean, or $E(\overline{X})$, is the mean of a normal distribution; the expected value of a proportion, or $E(p)$, is the mean of a binomial distribution, and the expected value of a very small proportion/rate, or $E(r)$, is the mean of a Poisson distribution. Cumulative incidence and prevalence rates may be either large or small proportions and therefore may be labeled either p *or* r. Coming from one of the distributions in the exponential family, all of the sample means, proportions, and rates we report in public health are calculated in the same way:

$$E(\overline{X}) = \mu \quad \text{and} \quad \overline{X} = \frac{\sum_{i=1}^{n} X_i}{n}$$

$$E(p) = \pi \quad \text{and} \quad p = \frac{\sum_{i=1}^{n} X_i}{n}$$

$$E(r) = \lambda \quad \text{and} \quad r = \frac{\sum_{i=1}^{n} X_i}{n}$$

Because means, proportions, and rates are unbiased estimates, the term for bias in the equation for accuracy equals 0 and drops out of the formula. It can then be rewritten as:

$$Accuracy = Reliability$$

The equation cannot be reduced any further, because even with zero bias, it is extremely unlikely that a statistic from one sample will exactly equal the population value. The reliability of an estimate, though, can and should always be assessed directly.

In order to evaluate the reliability of an observed statistic, we need to have a measure of the theoretical variability of all such statistics that might have been observed with infinite repeated sampling of the population. Remember that the variability of the values in the one sample we observe is measured by the familiar standard deviation (the square root of the variance):

$$\text{Standard Deviation of } X = S = \sqrt{\frac{\sum_{i=1}^{n}(X_I - \overline{X})^2}{n-1}}$$

The theoretical variability of statistics that summarize these values is then measured by what is called the standard error. The formulas for the *standard error* of means, proportions, and rates are:

$$\text{Normal}: \text{s.e.}(\overline{X}) = \frac{S}{\sqrt{n}} = \sqrt{\frac{\frac{\sum_{i=1}^{n}(X_i - \overline{X})^2}{n-1}}{n}}$$

$$\text{Binomial}: \text{s.e.}(p) = \sqrt{\frac{p(1-p)}{n}}$$

$$\text{Poisson}: \text{s.e.}(r) = \sqrt{\frac{r}{n}}$$

These formulas for the standard errors of means, proportions, and rates are not identical, but because the distributions of statistics belong to the same mathematical family they are analogous under certain circumstances (although the conventional notation is somewhat different). The standard error of the mean of a normal distribution is approximately equivalent to the standard error of a binomial proportion, and when proportions are very small, the standard error of a Poisson variable is also approximately equivalent as well.

$$\sqrt{\frac{\frac{\sum_{i=1}^{n}(X_i - \overline{X})^2}{n-1}}{n}} \cong \sqrt{\frac{p(1-p)}{n}} \cong \sqrt{\frac{r}{n}}$$

Returning to the example of number of well child visits, the standard error of the sample mean of 6.2 is calculated as follows:

$$\sqrt{\dfrac{\dfrac{(8-6.2)^2+(2-6.2)^2+(5-6.2)^2 \; \ldots \; +(9-6.2)^2+(6-6.2)^2+(3-6.2)^2}{19}}{20}}$$

$$=\dfrac{\text{standard deviation of the observed values}}{\sqrt{20}}=\dfrac{3.43}{\sqrt{20}}=0.77$$

Next, the standard error for the sample proportion of 0.30 with < 5 well child visits is calculated as follows:

$$\sqrt{\dfrac{0.30\times 0.70}{20}}$$

$$=0.102$$

Now, to illustrate the similarity between the formulas for the standard errors of means and proportions, the standard error for the sample proportion of 0.30 is recalculated using the formula for a normally distributed continuous variable. The 20 values are coded "1" for < 5 visits and "0" for >= 5 visits. The standard error is then calculated as follows:

$$\sqrt{\dfrac{\dfrac{(0-0.30)^2+(1-0.30)^2+(0-0.30)^2+\ldots+(0-0.30)^2+(0-0.30)^2+(1-0.30)^2}{19}}{20}}$$

$$=0.105$$

You can see that the results of 0.102 and 0.105 from the two calculations are very close.

Next, to illustrate when the binomial and Poisson formulas are equivalent, remember that many rates are measures of rare events and that this is exactly the circumstance in which the binomial distribution and the Poisson distribution become essentially interchangeable.

For example, suppose County A has 11 infant deaths out of a total of 1,375 live births. We've already shown that the risk of infant mortality, or the cumulative incidence rate, is 11/1,375=0.008, and that this closely approximates the true incidence density. This is a very small proportion compared to the 0.30 for our example of the proportion of children at age two with < 5 well child visits. When p is very small, then $(1-p)$ will be very close to 1, and the formula for the standard error for a binomial proportion reduces to that for a Poisson variable:

$$\sqrt{\dfrac{p(1-p)}{n}}\cong\sqrt{\dfrac{p(1)}{n}}\cong\sqrt{\dfrac{r}{n}}$$

The standard error for the infant mortality rate in County A is:

$$\sqrt{\frac{0.008 \times 0.992}{1,375}} \cong \sqrt{\frac{0.008 \times 1}{1,375}} \cong \sqrt{\frac{0.008}{1,375}}$$

$$= 0.0024$$

The similarity between the formulas for standard errors is easy to see when proportions are left in their decimal representations, but more typically, proportions are multiplied by a constant such as 100, 1,000, 10,000, or 100,000 to get the percents and rates in an integer form that is easier to interpret. The multipliers can either be applied after carrying out calculations, or they can be incorporated into the calculations from the start. The formulas for the standard errors of percents and rates can be rewritten as follows:

$$\text{Binomial}: \text{s.e.}(\%) = \sqrt{\frac{\%(100 - \%)}{n}}$$

$$\text{Poisson}: \text{s.e.}(\text{rate}) = \sqrt{\frac{\text{rate}}{n}} \times \text{multiplier}$$

$$\text{where multiplier} = 1,000, 10,000, 100,000$$

The standard error for the estimate of 30 % (as opposed to 0.30) with < 5 well child visits, then, becomes $0.012 \times 100 = 10.2$, and the standard error for the estimate of an infant mortality rate of 8 per 1,000 (as opposed to 0.008) in County A becomes $0.0024 \times 1,000 = 2.4$.

Question:

What distribution is appropriate for calculating the standard errors of the following statistics?

The C-section rate in County X is 18.3 per 100 deliveries
The average length of stay following delivery is 52.5 hours
The CSHCN program coverage rate is 67.3 per 100 eligible children
The homicide rate of children 0-3 is 3.9 per 100,000 children age 0-3

Answer:

binomial, normal, binomial, Poisson

The Central Limit Theorem

One of the most fundamental concepts from statistical theory is the *Central Limit Theorem*, which states that with relatively large sample size the distribution of summary statistics will be close to normal regardless of the original distribution of the values from which they were calculated. For example, while a relatively rare event such as infant death is assumed to follow a Poisson distribution, a set of hypothetical infant mortality rates from repeated sampling will approach being normally distributed. Each statistic we report, however, is distributed according to its own normal distribution with values corresponding to the scale on which it was measured. For instance, a program coverage rate might range from 30%-80%, the mean number of well child visits by age two might range from 3-12 visits, and infant mortality rates might range from 5-20 per 1,000 live births.

Determining probabilities for these distinct normal distributions that result from variables being measured on different scales is for all practical purposes impossible. Each distribution, though, can be rescaled to conform with the values of the *standard* normal distribution (z values) such that the mean of the new distribution is 0 with a standard deviation of 1. The standard normal distribution is powerful because it provides a unifying method for evaluating the accuracy of statistics.

Confidence Intervals

In addition to calculating a precise estimate of the standard error for a mean, proportion, or rate, we can assess the reliability of the statistics we report by estimating a range of values which includes the unknown population value with a given probability. This range is called a *confidence interval*, and by convention, 95 % confidence intervals are routinely calculated, although sometimes an interval with greater or less probability of containing the population value is appropriate. A narrow confidence interval indicates that the population value is probably quite close to the sample estimate; a wide confidence interval indicates that the population value may be quite far from the sample estimate.

In order to generate a confidence interval, points on a probability distribution are needed to define an area or range that contains the chosen amount of probability. To define the appropriate range, we use what are called critical values. These are usually taken from the standard normal distribution whether the confidence interval is for a mean, proportion, or a rate. On this scale, 95 % of the probability is contained between z values of -1.96 and +1.96. These are the critical values most widely used for calculating confidence limits.

Standard Normal Distribution

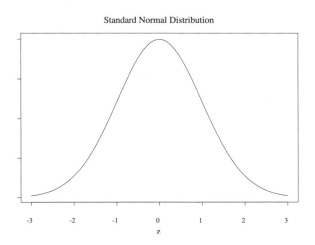

z

Even though the probability distributions in the exponential family have much in common, they are not interchangeable. The Central Limit Theorem does not apply as the size of the sample decreases; when sample size is very small it is necessary to use exact critical values from the t, binomial, or Poisson distribution rather than assuming that those from the standard normal curve are appropriate for estimating variability. Critical values for the distributions in the exponential family and their associated probabilities can be found in tables in most statistics and epidemiology textbooks. Even with larger sample size when critical values from the standard normal distribution can be used for calculating confidence intervals, the standard errors are calculated using the formulas for the distribution that best fits the data in order to maximize precision in evaluating the reliability of statistics.

Comment

For means, the rule of thumb is that 30 observations are needed in order to use z values. For proportions, the rule of thumb is that the number of observations multiplied by the proportion (or the number of events) should equal at least 5. This means that as proportions get smaller, the sample size requirements get larger. For example, if an infant mortality rate is 10 per 1,000 live births, then critical values from the standard normal curve can be used if there are at least 5 infant deaths or 500 live births ($0.010 \times 500 = 5$).

The general form of a confidence interval is:

$$\text{Upper Limit} = \text{Estimate} + \text{Critical Value} \times \text{Standard Error}$$

$$\text{Lower Limit} = \text{Estimate} + \text{Critical Value} \times \text{Standard Error}$$

To construct 95 % confidence intervals for the mean number of well child visits and the proportion of two-year-olds with < 5 well child visits from the sample of size 20, and for the infant mortality rate based on County A's 1,375 live births, we use the critical value 1.96:

Mean # of well child visits: $CI = 6.2 \pm 1.96 \times 0.77 = (4.7 \text{ - } 7.7)$

Proportion with < 5 visits: $CI = 30 \pm 1.96 \times 10.2 = (9.9 \text{ - } 50.1)$

Infant Mortality Rate: $CI = 8 \pm 1.96 \times 2.4 = (3.3 \text{ - } 12.7)$

Notice that in each of these calculations, 1.96 is used as the critical value for determining 95% probability, but that the standard errors are calculated using the formulas for means, proportions, and rates respectively.

Comment

Sometimes it is useful to calculate a confidence interval around the count of a rare event such as infant death. Particularly at the local level, reporting counts rather than rates may be preferable since they connect more concretely to the health experience of individuals. Let d = the count of infant deaths, and then the formula for the confidence interval around the rate can be algebraically transformed to yield a confidence interval around d:

$$CI(r) = r \pm 1.96\sqrt{\frac{r}{n}}$$

$$= \frac{d}{n} \pm 1.96\sqrt{\frac{d/n}{n}}$$

Once r has been transformed to d/n, a confidence interval around d can by calculated by multiplying each term by n:

$$CI(d) = n \times \frac{d}{n} \pm 1.96\sqrt{n^2 \times \frac{d}{n^2}}$$

$$= d \pm 1.96\sqrt{d}$$

For the 11 infant deaths in County A, the confidence interval is: $11 \pm 1.96\sqrt{11} = (4.5 - 17.5)$

To see the effect of sample size on the confidence interval, let's recalculate the interval around the estimate of 30 % of children with fewer than five well child visits assuming a sample size of 1,375 like that for County A's infant mortality rate. The standard error now becomes:

$$\sqrt{\frac{30 \times 70}{1,375}}$$

$$= 1.24$$

And the new confidence interval is: $CI = 30 \pm 1.96 \times 1.24 = (27.6 - 32.4)$

The narrowness of this interval based on a sample size of 1,375 compared to that when the estimate of 30 % is based on a sample size of 20 shows that we have much more confidence that our estimate is near to the population value—the estimate is said to be more reliable or more stable, and it is therefore more accurate.

Comment

Statistical software (or even hand calculators) cannot differentiate between a data-set containing values for individuals (individual) and one containing values for groups (aggregate); sample size equals the number of records in the data-set regardless of its structure. In an aggregate data-set containing 100 records, for example, if the data are not explicitly weighted according to the underlying population sizes (see comment and example on pages 22-25), confidence intervals around statistics will be computed using a sample size of 100. We know, however, that each of the hypothetical 100 counties has its own sample size, ranging, for instance, from 3,244 individuals to 2,988,653 individuals. Knowing the varying numbers of individuals on which the aggregate data are based is important for interpreting the county data and assessing potential error. Depending on the purpose of an analysis, assessment of the accuracy of estimates may use the sample size at the individual or at the aggregate level.

Question:

Calculate confidence intervals for the following statistics:

1. Mean length of stay following delivery of 52.5 hours, with a standard deviation of 26 hours and a sample size of 200.

2. CSHCN (children with special health care needs) program coverage rate of 67.3 % based on a sample size of 800

Answer:

1.
$$CI = 52.5 \pm 1.96 \times \frac{26}{\sqrt{200}}$$

$$= 52.5 \pm 3.6$$

$$= (49 - 56)$$

2.
$$CI = 67.3 \pm 1.96 \sqrt{\frac{67.3 \times 32.7}{800}}$$

$$= 67.3 \pm 3.25$$

$$= (64.1 - 70.6)$$

Choosing the Best Estimates

Often, we have several sources of information for variables that we wish to report; perhaps one statistic comes from a local survey while another comes from vital records. Different samples or data sources may contain estimates that are statistically biased or unbiased, and that are based on different sample or population sizes. The decision as to which estimate to report should be based on its accuracy:

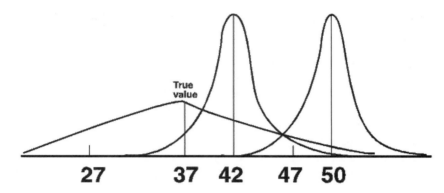

From Sampling of Populations: Methods and Applications, Paul S. Levy and Stanley Lemeshow. Copyright © 1991 by John Wiley & Sons, Inc. Used by permission of John Wiley & Sons, Inc.

One estimate is theoretically unbiased, but unreliable
One estimate is theoretically slightly biased, but very reliable
One estimate is theoretically very biased, but very reliable

Which is the best estimate?

As already pointed out, we use means, proportions, and rates because they are unbiased estimates of population values and so we can evaluate their accuracy simply by calculating standard errors to obtain confidence limits that measure their reliability. It is sometimes useful and necessary, however, to use other kinds of estimates which cannot be shown to be unbiased. Synthetic estimates, (see Module 3 for more details) for example, may contain bias and evaluation of their accuracy must take this into account.

Of course, the goal is to have an estimate that is both unbiased and very reliable, but often we are confronted with the situation illustrated in the above picture and we are forced to choose from among less than ideal statistics. Whatever we choose, evaluating the accuracy of statistics and presenting confidence limits for them is a step in information-based decision-making.

THE EPIDEMIOLOGIC VIEW OF BEST ESTIMATES

The ability to choose the best estimate goes beyond considerations of statistical bias and reliability. Epidemiology addresses the accuracy of estimates from the point of view of measurement rather than sampling theory. It adds more precise terminology and definitions for estimating the frequency and distribution of health and disease, focuses attention on how a variable should be defined, and evaluates measurement biases.

In addition to the points discussed earlier with regard to choices for categorizing variables, consideration must be given to potential biases, other than statistical bias in our data. The primary biases of concern stem from two phenomena: collecting information from a select population or inaccurate measurement of variables.

Biases Due to Collecting Information from a Select Population

Selection Bias. Often our estimates of a health event or outcome are not based on the entire population or a random sample of the entire population, but rather are based on a restricted group for whom we have data, either because of their willingness to respond to a survey, their ability to participate in a program, or because of a convenient opportunity to access data for these particular individuals. For example, it is possible that a survey of working mothers' day care choices is answered disproportionately by families in which the mother works part-time because the full-time working mothers are too busy to respond. The estimate of the frequency of type of day care choice derived from this survey would over-represent the practices of part-time mothers, not providing an accurate representation of the day care experiences of all working mothers.

Survivor Bias. One particular type of selection bias is *survivor bias*; this is a bias that results from obtaining information only from those who have survived to provide it. Survivor bias is common in perinatal epidemiology when estimates of pregnancy related risk factors and outcomes are based on data for live births rather than on all pregnancies. An example of this phenomenon is when we obtain an estimate of smoking behavior during pregnancy from women who have had live births and not from women who have had induced abortions, ectopic pregnancies, spontaneous abortions or fetal deaths. This will underestimate smoking prevalence during pregnancy if this behavior is more common among women whose pregnancies end in other than a live birth.

Biases Due to Measurement of Information

Often our estimates are biased because the information we obtain is inaccurate or incomplete. Sometimes we ask individuals to recall or document events that have occurred in the past. Because memory may fade the further one is from the occurrence of the event, or because memory may be influenced by the occurrence of an adverse health event, this information may be subject to *recall bias*. Another type of measurement bias occurs when we ask individuals to provide information on sensitive topics such as illicit substance use or certain sexual behaviors; as individuals seek to present themselves in the most favorable light, this information may be under-reported or even over-reported. Further, those responsible for documenting or recording information may differentially record events, procedures, or care experiences again leading to underreporting or over-reporting.

To illustrate one form of reporting bias, suppose that we know the true population value of an MCH indicator to be 9.9 %, and further suppose that by chance, both population data and survey data yield 10 % as an estimate of this value. Here, both estimates are unbiased statistically, but the narrow confidence interval around the population estimate indicates it is far more reliable and therefore far more accurate. Both confidence intervals, however, include 9.9 %.

	Estimate	n	s.e.
Population Data	10%	100,000	0.09
Survey Data	10%	100	3.00

$$CI_{pop} = 10 \pm 1.96(0.095) = (9.8 - 10.2)$$

$$CI_{surv} = 10 \pm 1.96(3.000) = (4.1 - 15.9)$$

Now suppose that the population data yields 5 % as an estimate while the survey data yields 10 % as an estimate. Both estimates are still statistically unbiased, but underreporting has biased the estimate from the population data and the reliability of the estimate is no longer meaningful since the confidence limit no longer even includes the true value of 9.9%. The estimate from the survey data, even with its wide confidence interval, is actually more accurate.

	Estimate	n	s.e.
Population Data	5%	100,000	0.07
Survey Data	10%	100	3.00

$$CI_{pop} = 5 \pm 1.96(0.07) = (4.9 - 5.1)$$

$$CI_{surv} = 10 \pm 1.96(3.00) = (4.1 - 15.9)$$

Due to inaccurate measurement we may also misclassify an individual as having or not having a particular risk factor/marker or outcome. Even though misclassification is never desirable, we can accept some amount of random misclassification. Our primary concern is systematic misclassification because this will be most likely to lead to either inflated or deflated estimates of association. *Random misclassification* means that all of the individuals for whom we have data are equally likely to be misclassified; *systematic misclassification* means that a particular group or groups of individuals have a greater chance of being misclassified than do others in the sample.

──Comment

Systematic misclassification occurs, for example, when women who obtain prenatal care from a provider who routinely fails to transfer prenatal care records to the hospital of delivery are classified as having had no prenatal care because there is no record to provide evidence of that care. Similarly, particular groups of women (e.g., low income women) may be more consistently classified as smokers or drug users because their prenatal care providers are more likely to ascertain and record this information. Misclassification of this type will lead to inaccurate estimates of statistics such as the percent of women with no prenatal care or the percent of women who smoke during pregnancy, and this in turn may lead to an underestimate or overestimate of the relationship between these variables and other risk factors or outcomes of interest.

Both statistical and epidemiological biases must be taken into account when choosing an appropriate estimate to report. Likewise, one may be forced to present the biased estimate but may want to present it with an acknowledgment of the ways in which it may not represent the true experience of the population of interest. The formula for the accuracy of estimates is again:

Accuracy = Bias + Reliability

where bias should be interpreted as encompassing both the statistical and epidemiological meaning.

Question:

What type of bias may be present in the following examples?

1. As part of designing an intervention program to reduce low birthweight, you discover that mothers of children with intrauterine growth retardation (IUGR) report greater caffeine consumption in the first trimester of pregnancy than mothers of children without IUGR. Before you develop a significant anti-caffeine component for your program you decide to consider that some bias may be operating in these reports. What bias might be operative?

2. You are developing a program for children with cerebral palsy in several regions of the state and you receive very diverse prevalence estimates as well as differing risk factor profiles associated with cerebral palsy from your Children with Special Health Care Needs regional coordinators. You think that some biases may be leading to these varying estimates. What might these be?

3. You are developing a profile of asthma prevalence and morbidity among children in your county. Based on information obtained from hospital discharge data, you notice that some population groups appear to have a greater prevalence of hospitalizations for asthma. You are considering a press release to discuss the greater prevalence of asthma in these groups, and to call for more funding targeted at prevention and treatment programs for these groups. Before you release your report you discuss the findings with your agency director who reminds you of the possibility of bias. What bias might be operating?

Answer:

1. Recall bias—a type of information bias in which groups differentially report events of the past dependent on their current health status outcomes may be present. Mothers of children with IUGR may search harder in their memories for a potential "cause" of this adverse perinatal outcome.

2. Survivor bias, a type of selection bias, as well as information bias may be present. If the risk factor profiles are based on children diagnosed with cerebral palsy at the age of two, they reflect those of the "survivors" which may be different than if the profiles were based on children diagnosed earlier (survivor bias). In addition, prevalence estimates of cerebral palsy will differ depending on the timing of case ascertainment (information bias) because many early neurological deficits will disappear by the age of two and other nonspecific motor signs may evolve over the first year or two into spasticity. There may also be a systematic recording difference between counties that needs to be investigated (information bias).

3. Selection bias may be present. Children who are hospitalized for asthma are more likely to be those who are low-income, uninsured, or from more vulnerable families, and more likely to experience more severe asthma episodes as a result of inability to access the primary care delivery system. By examining only hospital cases, an accurate assessment of asthma prevalence as well as an authentic profile of risk factors associated with childhood asthma cannot be produced.

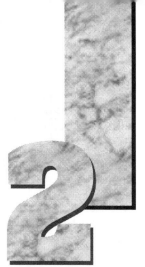

Measures of Association and Hypothesis Testing

by Deborah Rosenberg, PhD and Arden Handler, DrPH

Once best estimates are chosen, both from a statistical and epidemiologic perspective, hypotheses about the estimated association between a single mean, proportion, or rate and a fixed value, typically a standard or goal, or about the estimated association between two or more means, proportions, or rates can be tested. Hypotheses address questions about whether any observed differences in health status, risk and protective factors, health services or health systems indicators are real or spurious.

Statistics to test hypotheses take the following general form:

$$\text{Test Statistic} = \frac{\text{Observed Association - Expected Association}}{\text{Standard Error of the Association}}$$

Here, the observed association is the comparison of a single estimate and a standard or the comparison of two or more estimates, and the expected association reflects the same comparison but under what is called the *null hypothesis* or the assumption that no association exists.

Observed associations and the test statistics used for evaluating them follow known probability distributions. Critical values can be chosen to assess the probability that the observed association is different from its expected value. As with single means, proportions, or rates, measures of association are statistically unbiased estimates of the true population experience. They estimate average association just as single measures estimate average occurrence.

There are two types of error that can be made when testing hypotheses:

Type I Error: Concluding that there is an association when one does not exist
Type II Error: Concluding that there is no association when one does exist

The probability of interpreting an observed association as real when it is in fact due to chance, or the probability of committing a Type I error, is what is reported as the p-value.

By convention, associations are considered statistically significant when the p-value is < 0.05, although other values are also used depending on the analysis. Since, as we've already seen, 95% of the probability in the standard normal distribution lies between -1.96 and 1.96, these are typically chosen as critical values. Any result from a statistical test based on the standard normal curve which is less than -1.96 or greater than 1.96 means that there is less than a 5% probability (p < 0.05) that observed differences are due to chance alone.

In addition to using p-values, confidence limits can also be calculated around measures of association. These confidence limits define a range of values within which the true population association is likely to lie, and tell us about the reliability of our data.

The confidence intervals for many measures of association take the general form:

$$CI = \text{Observed Association} \pm \text{Critical Value} \times \text{Standard Error of the Association}$$

MEASURES OF ASSOCIATION: DIFFERENCE MEASURES

Differences between means, proportions, and rates can theoretically range from negative infinity to positive infinity ($-\infty$ to ∞), with their expected values, assuming no association, being 0. In other words, one of the means (or proportions) being compared may theoretically be either infinitely less than or infinitely greater than the other one, and if the two means (or proportions) are equal, then the difference between them will be 0. The distribution of a difference measure is approximately normal if sample size is reasonably large. Statistical testing, therefore, can usually rely on the known values of the standard normal curve.

Two Independent Means

For two independent means, the measure of association is their observed difference:

$$\overline{X}_1 - \overline{X}_2$$

The expected association under the null hypothesis is that $\overline{X}_1 - \overline{X}_2 = 0$. Then, the formula that gives a test of statistical significance follows the t distribution, a generalization of the normal distribution, as follows:

$$t = \frac{\overline{X}_1 - \overline{X}_2 - 0}{\sqrt{\frac{(n_1 - 1)S_1^2 + (n_2 - 1)S_2^2}{n_1 + n_2 - 2}\left(\frac{1}{n_1} + \frac{1}{n_2}\right)}}$$

where S is the standard deviation of the observed values

Here, the observed value is the actual difference between the two means and the expected value is 0 under the null hypothesis. The standard error of the measure of association is the sum of the standard errors of the two means being compared. Assuming that the two variances are actually the same as shown above, a common variance can be estimated by taking the average of the two sample variances in the data, weighted by the number of observations contributing to each mean.

The formula for the confidence interval around the difference between two independent means is as follows:

$$\left(\overline{X}_1 - \overline{X}_2\right) \pm 1.96 \sqrt{\frac{S_1^2}{n_1} + \frac{S_2^2}{n_2}}$$

Now the formula for the standard error is slightly different than that used for the statistical test. When calculating confidence limits, we are simply estimating the error around the observed association without any reference to a null hypothesis, and therefore the constraint of a common variance imposed on the statistical test does not apply. Here, the standard error is simply the unweighted sum of the variances of the two means being compared.

Suppose we want to compare the mean number of well child visits received by children in the first two years of life in two counties. The mean in County A is observed to be 6.2 with a standard deviation of 3.4 (square root of the variance) based on a sample of 200 two-year-olds. The mean in County B is observed to be 5.3 with a standard deviation of 4.5 based on a sample of 150 two-year-olds. On average, are the children in the two counties receiving the same amount of well child care? The test statistic to estimate the answer to this question is:

$$t = \frac{(6.2 - 5.3) - 0}{\sqrt{\frac{199 \times 3.4^2 + 149 \times 4.5^2}{200 + 150 - 2} \left(\frac{1}{200} + \frac{1}{150}\right)}}$$

$$= \frac{0.9 - 0}{\sqrt{15.3 \left(\frac{1}{200} + \frac{1}{150}\right)}}$$

$$= \frac{0.9}{0.42} = 2.1$$

The common variance is 15.3, or a standard deviation of 3.9, a weighted average of the standard deviations of 3.4 in County A and 4.5 in County B. The weights are the proportion of the total sample contributed by each county—57% $((199/348) \times 100)$ for County A and 43% $((149/348) \times 100)$ for County B.

The result of 2.1 tells us that the observed difference in the two means is slightly more than 2 standard deviations away from the expected difference of 0. According to the values on the standard normal curve (equivalent to the t distribution with this sample size), there is only a 2% probability of seeing this test result or one even farther away from 0 if, in fact, the two-year-olds in County A and County B are receiving the same number of well child visits on average. In other words, it is very unlikely ($p \cong 0.02$) that the difference we observe is due solely to chance. Since 2.1 > 1.96, we report that County A's mean is significantly different than County B's ($p < 0.05$).

The confidence interval around the difference between the two means is:

$$CI = (6.2 - 5.3) \pm 1.96 \sqrt{\frac{3.4^2}{200} + \frac{4.5^2}{150}}$$

$$= 0.9 \pm 1.96 \sqrt{0.19}$$

$$= 0.9 \pm 0.85$$

$$= (0.05 - 1.75)$$

Since the confidence interval of 0.05-1.75 does not include the expected value of 0, the two means are shown to be statistically different.

Two Independent Proportions

For two proportions, there are several measures of association that can be examined. Epidemiology uses the 2×2 table as the framework for constructing these measures:

Disease or Other Health Outcome

		Yes	No	
	Yes	a	b	a + b (n_1)
Exposure or Person, Place, or Time Characteristic	No	c	d	c + d (n_2)
		a + c (m_1)	b + d (m_2)	a + b + c + d N

Comment

If the proportions are incidence density data, the 2×2 table is actually slightly different than above because the denominators are not counts of individuals; n_1 and n_2 are person-time data and therefore quantities for cells b and d cannot be calculated. Public health data, however, are typically cumulative incidence or prevalence data, and so the focus will be on the 2×2 table as shown in the above figure.

For the moment, we will assume that the data in the 2×2 table are either complete population data or data from a random sample. In other words, N is the population or sample total, n_1 and n_2 are the population or sample totals of those with and without the exposure, and m_1 and m_2 are the population or sample totals of those with and without the disease. These are the kind of data typically encountered by public health agencies for use in surveillance and monitoring. Later, we will discuss changes in the 2×2 table when data are not population data or data from a random sample, but are instead from more complex sampling designs used in some surveys and research studies.

Notice, that for public health purposes, the exposure variable in the 2×2 table may be a medical risk factor, a social or behavioral risk factor, a person characteristic, the place of occurrence, the time of occurrence, or a person-place-time characteristic. The health status outcome variable may be a disease, a behavior, a measure of access to care or service utilization, or any other measure that is hypothesized to be an outcome of the "exposure". In addition, the 2×2 table can be used to examine data derived from ecologic analyses in which information is for exposures and outcomes for groups rather than individuals (e.g., percent uninsured in each area and % of children with asthma in each area). The framework of the 2 × 2 table accommodates data from a wide variety of sources and is a valuable tool for organizing data for a wide variety of analyses.

Examples of 2 × 2 Tables

1. Individual Level Data on a Risk Factor and a Health Outcome

		Health Outcome		
		Yes	No	
Smoking	Yes	a	b	n_1
	No	c	d	n_2
		m_1	m_2	N individuals

2. Individual Level Data on a Person Characteristic and a Health Outcome

		Health Outcome		
		Yes	No	
Low	Yes	a	b	n_1
Income	No	c	d	n_2
		m_1	m_2	N individuals

3. Individual Level Data on Place of Residence and a Health Outcome

		Health Outcome		
		Yes	No	
Residence	County A	a	b	n_1
	County B	c	d	n_2
		m_1	m_2	N individuals

4. Individual Level Data on Time of Occurrence and a Health Outcome

		Health Outcome		
		Yes	No	
Occurrence	Time 1	a	b	n_1
	Time 2	c	d	n_2
		m_1	m_2	N individuals

5. Individual Level Data on a Person-Place-Time Characteristic and a Health Outcome

		Health Outcome		
		Yes	No	
Residence in	Yes	a	b	n_1
Low-Income Area	No	c	d	n_2
		m_1	m_2	N individuals

6. Ecologic Analysis
Aggregate Level Data on a Risk Factor and a Health Outcome

		Health Outcome		
		% High	% Low	
% Smokers	> 20 %	a	b	n_1
in Area	<=20%	c	d	n_2
		m_1	m_2	N areas

7. Ecologic Analysis
Aggregate Level Data on a Person-Place-Time Characteristic and a Health Outcome

		Health Outcome		
		% High	% Low	
% Low-Income	> 20 %	a	b	n_1
in Area	<= 20%	c	d	n_2
		m_1	m_2	N areas

Comment

An important distinction must be made between ecologic variables and ecologic analysis. Table 5 above illustrates what we have termed a person-place-time variable, or a person characteristic aggregated in units of geography and time. Person-place-time variables are examples of ecologic variables. The variables "residence in a low income community" or "percent low-income in the community" have values that can be assigned to each individual in a sample, although the information they contain pertains to the environment within which the individual lives. Risk factor and outcome variables can also be ecologic variables if they are aggregates in time and place. For example, "prevalence of smoking among women giving birth in a community", "county prevalence of unintended pregnancy", or "city infant mortality rate" are ecologic variables with values that can be assigned to individuals.

A data-set in which the observations, or units of analysis, are unique individuals may contain a mixture of individual level variables and ecologic variables. For example, values for smoking status during pregnancy and delivery of a low birthweight infant, as well as values for the smoking prevalence among women delivering in the individual's county and the low birthweight rate in the individual's county might be collected for each individual. The data for five individuals from a hypothetical MCH individual level data-set might look like:

Individual	Variables			
	Smoking during pregnancy	Infant Birthweight < 2500 grams	Smoking Prevalence in Community	Low Birthweight Prevalence in Community
1	Yes	No	15 %	8%
2	No	Yes	10 %	6%
3	No	No	20 %	10%
4	Yes	Yes	20 %	9%
5	No	No	15 %	7%

Including ecologic variables in an analysis of individuals is not equivalent to conducting an ecologic analysis. In an ecologic analysis, the observations in the data-set, or units of analysis, are either geographic areas, health facilities, schools, time periods, or other aggregates. No data for individuals are available. Instead, analysis is focused on the relationship between exposure and outcome for the groups in the data-set and not directly on the individuals they encompass.

The data for five communities from a hypothetical aggregate level MCH data-set might look like:

Community	Variables	
	Smoking Prevalence in Community	Low Birthweight Prevalence in Community
1	15 %	8%
2	10 %	6%
3	20 %	10%
4	20 %	9%
5	15 %	7%

Analogous to the measure of association for two means, comparison of two proportions may also be evaluated using a difference measure:

$$\frac{a}{n_1} - \frac{c}{n_2} = p_1 - p_2 \text{ or } r_1 - r_2$$

And the test of statistical significance can either be in a form that follows the χ^2 or the z (standard normal) distribution:

	Outcome		
	Yes	No	
Risk Yes	a	b	n_1
Factor No	c	d	n_2
	m_1	m_2	N

$$\chi^2 = \sum_{i=a}^{d} \frac{(O_i - E_i)^2}{E_i}$$

where O_i = the observed value in each cell   or

and $E_i = \dfrac{\text{row total} \times \text{column total}}{N}$

$$z = \frac{(p_1 - p_2) - 0}{\sqrt{p_0(1 - p_0)\left(\dfrac{1}{n_1} + \dfrac{1}{n_2}\right)}}$$

With the Poisson assumption for rates, the formula can be rewritten:

$$z = \frac{r_1 - r_2 - 0}{\sqrt{r_0\left(\dfrac{1}{n_1} + \dfrac{1}{n_2}\right)}}$$

For the z tests, p_1 and $r_1 = \dfrac{a}{n_1}$, p_2 and $r_2 = \dfrac{c}{n_2}$, and p_0 and $r_0 = \dfrac{m_1}{N}$

The formula using the chi-square distribution compares the observed and expected value of the counts in each cell of the 2 × 2 table, while the z test compares the observed and expected value of the difference in proportions. The two tests are equivalent; that is, for the 2 × 2 table, $\chi^2 = z^2$. The p-values associated with these two tests are also equivalent and therefore the conclusions drawn will be identical.

As in the t test for means, the observed value in the z test is the actual difference between the two proportions and the expected value is 0 under the null hypothesis. The standard error of the measure of association is the sum of the standard errors of the proportions being compared. Assuming that the two variances are actually the same, a common variance can be estimated by taking the average of the two sample variances in the data, weighted by the number of observations contributing to each proportion.

The formulas for calculating confidence intervals around the difference between two independent proportions are:

$$\text{Binomial}: \text{CI} = p_1 - p_2 \pm 1.96\sqrt{\frac{p_1(1 - p_1)}{n_1} + \frac{p_2(1 - p_2)}{n_2}}$$

$$\text{Poisson}: \text{CI} = r_1 - r_2 \pm 1.96\sqrt{\frac{r_1}{n_1} + \frac{r_2}{n_2}}$$

Once again, the formulas for the standard errors are somewhat different than for the statistical tests because the null hypothesis is not being tested.

Comment

In practice, the formula for the standard error which simply sums the variances of the means or proportions being compared is often used for calculating test statistics as well as for confidence intervals. This is a reasonable approach since the results of using this formula and those from using the one requiring estimation of a common variance are usually very similar.

Let's return to the example of County A with its infant mortality rate of 8 per 1,000 based on 1,375 live births. Suppose that County B has an infant mortality rate of 6.7 based on 900 births. On average, is the infant mortality experience in these two counties different? Below is the 2 × 2 table to examine these data more carefully:

		Infant Death		
		Yes	No	
County	A	11	1,364	1,375
	B	6	894	900
		17	2,258	2,275

We can use the χ^2 formula for testing the difference between these two rates. In order to do this we first need to calculate the expected values for each cell in the table:

$$E_1 = \frac{17 \times 1,375}{2,275} = 10.3, \quad E_2 = \frac{2,258 \times 1,375}{2,275} = 1,364.7$$

$$E_3 = \frac{17 \times 900}{2,275} = 6.7, \quad E_2 = \frac{2,258 \times 900}{2,275} = 893.3$$

Then the test statistic to estimate whether County A and County B have different infant mortality rates is:

$$\chi^2 = \frac{(11 - 10.3)^2}{10.3} + \frac{(1,364 - 1,364.7)^2}{1,364.7} + \frac{(6 - 6.7)^2}{6.7} + \frac{(894 - 893.3)^2}{893.3}$$

$$= 0.7^2 \left(\frac{1}{10.3} + \frac{1}{1,364.7} + \frac{1}{6.7} + \frac{1}{893.3} \right)$$

$$= 0.12$$

We can also use the standard normal distribution to test the difference between the two rates. Since these are cumulative incidence rates of a fairly rare event (infant death), we will use the formula with the Poisson assumption. In order to do this we first need to calculate the estimate of the common variance (r_0) that, in this example, is the overall infant mortality rate for both counties combined:

$$\frac{m_1}{N} \times 1{,}000 = \frac{17}{2{,}275} \times 1{,}000 = 7.5$$

Then the test statistic to estimate whether County A and County B have different infant mortality rates is:

$$z = \frac{8 - 6.7 - 0}{\sqrt{7.5\left(\frac{1}{1{,}375} + \frac{1}{900}\right)} \times 1{,}000}$$

$$= 0.35$$

Remember that since the two rates are in
integer form (8 and 6.7) rather than decimal form (0.008 and 0.0067),
we need to use the multiplier of 1,000 in the denominator.

And 0.35^2, or z^2, $= 0.12$, the same as the chi-square value we obtained above.

The result of 0.35 means that the observed difference in the two rates is much less than 1 standard deviation away from the expected difference of 0. According to the values on the standard normal curve, there is a 73% probability of seeing this test result or one even farther away from 0 if, in fact, the infant mortality experience in County A and County B is actually the same on average. In other words, it is very likely ($p \cong 0.73$) that the difference we observe is due solely to chance. Since $0.35 < 1.96$, we report that County A's infant mortality rate is not significantly different than County B's ($p > 0.05$).

The confidence limits around the difference in the two infant mortality rates is:

$$CI = (8 - 6.7) \pm 1.96 \sqrt{\left(\frac{8}{1{,}375} + \frac{6.7}{900}\right) \times 1{,}000}$$

$$= 1.3 \pm 1.96\sqrt{13.26}$$

$$= 1.3 \pm 7.14$$

$$= (-5.8 - 8.4)$$

Since the confidence interval of −5.8-8.4 includes the expected value of 0, the county rates are not statistically different.

The Attributable Risk

The difference between two proportions is given a specific interpretation in epidemiology called the *attributable risk* (AR). The attributable risk quantifies the number of occurrences of a health outcome that are due to, or can be attributed to, the exposure or risk factor. In order for this interpretation to apply, the relationship between the risk factor and outcome must be hypothesized to be causal. Looking at a few examples will better illustrate this point.

Consider the association between smoking and low birthweight shown in the 2 × 2 table below:

		Low Birthweight		
		Yes	No	
Smoker	Yes	280	2,720	3,000
	No	720	11,280	12,000
		1,000	14,000	15,000

The proportion of smokers who deliver low birthweight infants is 280/3,000 or 9.33% and the proportion of non-smokers who deliver low birthweight infants is 720/12,000 or 6.0%. The difference between these two proportions, or the attributable risk is:

$$\text{Attributable Risk} = p_1 - p_2 = 9.33 - 6.0 = 3.33$$

Comment

The test of statistical significance for the difference between these 2 binomial proportions is:

$$z = \frac{9.33 - 6.0}{\sqrt{6.67 \times 93.33 \left(\frac{1}{3,000} + \frac{1}{12,000} \right)}} = 6.5$$

which is highly significant (p<0.0001) since 6.5 is much greater than the critical value of 1.96.

The attributable risk defines the excess risk of delivering a low birthweight infant among the *group with the risk factor* of interest, in this case the women who smoke. For this example, 3.33 out of every 100 live births to smokers are infants whose low birthweight can be attributed to smoking.

From a public health perspective, it is often more useful to re-define the attributable risk in terms of the *whole population*, in this case all live births regardless of whether their mothers smoke. This modified measure is called the population attributable risk (PAR).

Instead of comparing the outcomes for those with and without a risk factor, as is done for statistical testing (and the AR), the PAR compares the outcomes for the whole population to those without the risk factor. In this example, the proportion of all women delivering who had a low birthweight infant is 1,000/15,000 or 6.67%, and, as we've already seen, the proportion of non-smokers delivering a low birthweight infant is 6.0%. The PAR is:

$$\text{Population Attributable Risk} = p_0 - p_2 = 6.67 - 6.0 = 0.67$$

Here the excess in low birthweight is expressed in terms of the experience of all live births. For this example, 0.67 out of every 100 live births are infants whose low birthweight can be attributed to smoking.

For both the attributable risk (AR) and the population attributable risk (PAR), the low birthweight percent among the non-smokers, or 6.0%, is considered the low birthweight percent expected among all live births if no women smoked during pregnancy. If the prevalence of smoking were reduced to 0, the 2 × 2 table would become a 1 × 2 table since there would no longer be any exposed group:

		Low Birthweight		
		Yes	No	
Smoking	No	900	14,100	15,000
		900	14,100	15,000

The 900 expected low birthweight infants in the table is arrived at by multiplying the expected population proportion of 0.06 by the 15,000 total live births:

$$0.06 \times 15,000 = 900$$

which is 100 fewer than the 1,000 low birthweight infants seen in the original 2 × 2 table. The 100 preventable low birthweight births can also be found directly by multiplying the AR by the number of smokers (0.0333 x 3,000=100), or by multiplying the PAR by the total number of live births (0.0067 x 15,000=100).

Thus far, we have used the attributable risk or the population attributable risk to assess the impact of completely eliminating a risk factor. The 2 × 2 table can also be used as a tool to examine the impact of reducing the prevalence of a risk factor to something more than 0. This fits a more realistic scenario in which a public health intervention might be able to reduce partially, though not completely, the prevalence of a risk factor.

In the smoking and low birthweight example, the observed prevalence of smoking is 20% (3,000/15,000), and from a public health perspective it would be important to estimate the impact of reducing this to, say, 15%. The numbers in the 2 × 2 table can be rearranged to conform to this hypothetical situation:

		Low Birthweight		
		Yes	No	
Smoker	Yes	210	2,040	2,250
	No	765	11,985	12,750
		975	14,025	15,000

The percent low birthweight among smokers and non-smokers has not been changed and neither, therefore, has the attributable risk which is still 3.33 per 100 births among the smokers. The number of low birthweight births, however, has dropped from 1,000 to 975, resulting in an overall low birthweight percent of 6.5. Only the prevalence of smoking has changed, from 20% (3,000/15,000) to 15% (2,250/15,000), and this 5% decrease means 25 fewer low birthweight births.

By having an impact on the prevalence of smoking among pregnant women, the population attributable risk has changed to:

$$\text{Population Attributable Risk} = p_0 - p_2 = 6.5 - 6.0 = 0.5$$

Now, only 0.5 out of every 100 births are infants whose low birthweight is attributed to smoking during pregnancy. The population attributable risk, then, is a function of the attributable risk and the prevalence of the risk factor in the population. It makes sense that as the prevalence of a risk factor decreases, the less of a contribution it makes to the overall occurrence (p_0) of an adverse outcome. The PAR can be rewritten as:

$$\text{Population Attributable Risk} = \text{Attributable Risk} \times \text{Prevalence of Risk}$$

$$p_0 - p_2 = (p_1 - p_2) \times \frac{n_1}{N}$$

For example:

$$6.67 - 6.0 = 3.33 \times 0.20 = 0.67$$

and following the reduction in smoking prevalence:

$$6.5 - 6.0 = 3.33 \times 0.15 = 0.50$$

Two other measures based on the attributable risk and the population attributable risk, are perhaps the most useful in describing the importance of a risk factor's contribution to an adverse outcome. These two measures are the attributable risk percent (AR%) and the population attributable risk percent (PAR%). The AR% simply converts the attributable risk into the percent of adverse outcomes preventable in the group with the risk factor, while the PAR% simply converts the population attributable risk into the percent of adverse outcomes preventable in the entire population at risk. The conversion into percents makes these measures more readily understandable and therefore more meaningful to report than the AR and PAR themselves.

Continuing with the smoking and low birthweight data, the formulas for the AR% and PAR% are:

$$\text{Attributable Risk } \% = \frac{p_1 - p_2}{p_1} \times 100 = \frac{3.33}{9.33} \times 100 = 36\%$$

$$\text{Population Attributable Risk } \% = \frac{p_0 - p_2}{p_0} \times 100 = \frac{0.67}{6.67} \times 100 = 10\%$$

Thirty-six percent of the low birthweight infants born to the 3,000 smokers may be attributable to smoking; 10% of the low birthweight infants born to the 15,000 pregnant women may be attributable to smoking.

Alternatively, from the 1 x 2 table that resulted when the prevalence of smoking was hypothetically reduced to 0, we saw that the number of low birthweight births was reduced by 100. The AR% is this number of potentially preventable adverse outcomes divided by the 280 smokers who delivered low birthweight infants (100/280=0.36) and the PAR% is this number of potentially preventable adverse outcomes divided by the total of 1,000 women who delivered low birthweight infants (100/1,000=10%).

The meaning of the attributable risk and its associated measures shifts when the exposure is not a risk factor. Suppose, instead of smoking, the rows of the 2 × 2 table with low birthweight are County A and County B. While it would be inappropriate to consider a county to be a cause of low birthweight, and therefore to attribute 3.3 low birthweight infants per 100 births directly to some feature of residence in County A, this value can be used to provide a practical interpretation to the significant statistical test results that were previously obtained. It might be fair to state that, on average, County A has an excess of 36% low birthweight births compared to County B.

Question:

Using the data below for the same population of 15,000 live births described above, calculate the attributable risk, the population attributable risk, the attributable risk % and the population attributable risk % for the association of cocaine use during pregnancy and low birthweight.

		Low Birthweight		
		Yes	No	
Cocaine	Yes	130	370	500
Use	No	870	13,630	14,500
		1,000	14,000	15,000

Answer:

LBW among cocaine users is 130/500 × 100 or 26% (p_1)
LBW among non-users is 870/14,500 × 100 or 6% (p_2)
Overall LBW is 1,000/15,000 × 100 or 6.67 % (p_0)

$$AR = 26.0 - 6.0 = 20.0$$

$$PAR = 6.67 - 6.0 = 0.67$$

$$AR\% = \frac{20.0}{26.0} \times 100 = 77\%$$

$$PAR\% = \frac{0.67}{6.67} \times 100 = 10\%$$

Note that the PAR and PAR% in this example are exactly the same as those calculated for the association between smoking and low birthweight in the same population. This is because, while cocaine use is a much more potent risk factor for low birthweight than smoking and therefore the cocaine AR and AR% are much higher, the prevalence of cocaine use is much lower than the prevalence of smoking. These two forces—the magnitude of the risk difference and the magnitude of the difference in prevalence—offset each other, leading to the same PAR and PAR%.

Hypotheses about a Mean, Proportion, or Rate in Comparison to a Standard

Thus far, excess risk, causal or otherwise, has been defined in terms of the observed proportion for the lower risk group. In the low birthweight example on page 57, the low birthweight percent in the non-smokers was, in effect, the expected value; in the infant mortality example on pages 55-56, the infant mortality rate in County B was, in effect, the expected value. Often, instead of defining the expected value in these terms, it is useful to use a standard. The standard might be the current level of an outcome in the nation or the state, or a national or state goal.

The test of significance for the difference between a proportion and a standard is:

$$z = \frac{p_1 - \text{Standard}}{\sqrt{\dfrac{\text{Standard}(1 - \text{Standard})}{n_1}}} \quad \text{or} \quad z = \frac{r_1 - \text{Standard}}{\sqrt{\dfrac{\text{Standard}}{n_1}}}$$

This formula is exactly the same as that for the difference between two proportions if we treat the standard as though it was a proportion from an infinite (or very large) population. With this assumption of extremely large sample size, the value of the standard dominates the overall proportion or rate, and its standard error equals (or approaches) 0. The formula for comparing two proportions, then, reduces to the one above. For example, comparing County A's infant mortality rate to the Year 2000 Objective of 7 per 1,000 live births, assuming the standard is based on a population of 10,000,000 live births, the data can be arranged in a 2 × 2 table as follows:

	Infant Death		
	Yes	No	
County A	11	1,364	1,375
Year 2000 Objective	70,000	9,930,000	10,000,000
	70,011	9,931,364	10,001,375

The equivalence of the test for two proportions (or two rates) with the test for a proportion (or rate) and a standard can now be shown. The following example is for the case of a Poisson variable (rate):

The formula for testing the difference between two rates is (see page 54)

$$\frac{8-7}{\sqrt{7\left(\dfrac{1}{1,375}+\dfrac{1}{10,000,000}\right)\times 1,000}}$$

and it reduces to the formula for testing the difference between one rate and a standard

$$\cong \frac{8-7}{\sqrt{\dfrac{7}{1,375}\times 1,000}}$$

$$=0.44$$

The overall proportion (70,011/10,001,375) is essentially equal to the standard, and the standard error of the standard (7/10,000,000) essentially equals 0. Similar to the results when comparing County A to County B (pages 55-56), the conclusion from this statistical test is that County A's rate is not different from the Year 2000 Objective; since 0.44 < 1.96, the critical value from the standard normal distribution.

Comment

If the standard to be used is not simply a goal, but actual data from the nation or the state, the comparison is technically not between two independent proportions since the data for the geographic area of interest is also data included in the standard. This violates one of the assumptions underlying the statistical test. When the estimates are not independent, the standard error of their difference will be underestimated by the usual calculation. On the other hand, the difference itself will be underestimated since the inclusion of the local data in the standard makes the standard and the local area more similar. These two errors—the underestimate of the standard error and the underestimate of the difference itself—may counteract each other, but the analyst must be aware of the potential for spurious results. If the population size of the geographic area of interest is much smaller than that of the standard, it is fairly safe to ignore the assumption of independence and proceed with statistical testing as usual.

Example

A statistical test of the difference between the 6.67% low birthweight seen previously in the hypothetical population of 15,000 live births and the Year 2000 Objective of 5 % is calculated as follows [for low birthweight, we use the formula for a binomial variable (percent)]:

$$z = \frac{6.67-5}{\sqrt{\dfrac{5.0(100-5.0)}{15,000}}}=9.6$$

Remember that since the proportion and the standard are in integer form (6.67 and 5) rather than decimal form (0.067 and 0.05), we need to use the multiplier of 100 in the denominator.

Since 9.6 is greater than the critical value of 1.96, the extent of low birthweight births in this population is significantly higher than the Year 2000 Objective. Because the sample size is large (15,000 live births), the estimate of 6.7% is very reliable and so we are quite confident that it is truly different from the goal of 5%. If this same test were carried out for a much smaller population of, say, 500 live births with the same estimate of 6.7 % low birthweight, the results would be:

$$z = \frac{6.67 - 5}{\sqrt{\frac{5.0(100 - 5.0)}{500}}} = 1.7$$

Since 1.7 is less than the critical value of 1.96, the extent of low birthweight births in this population is not shown to be significantly different than the Year 2000 Objective. Because the sample size is small (500 live births) and much less reliable than for the larger population, we are not as confident that the estimate of 6.67% is truly different from the goal of 5%.

MEASURES OF ASSOCIATION: RATIO MEASURES

The Relative Risk, The Relative Prevalence, and The Odds Ratio

In addition to the measures of association based on differences between means, proportions, or rates, epidemiology has contributed two measures of association based on ratios. The relative risk (RR) is the cumulative incidence in the exposed population divided by the cumulative incidence in the unexposed. When the data are based on prevalence rather than incidence, this measure is termed relative prevalence (RP). The relative risk and relative prevalence are calculated as follows:

$$RR \text{ and } RP = \frac{\frac{a}{a+b}}{\frac{c}{c+d}} = \frac{\frac{a}{n_1}}{\frac{c}{n_2}} = \frac{r_1}{r_2} \text{ or } \frac{p_1}{p_2}$$

The other measure contributed by epidemiology, the *odds ratio*, is the odds of having the outcome in the exposed divided by the odds of having the outcome in the unexposed. The odds ratio does not use the population denominators of n_1 and n_2, but just the numbers in the cells of the 2 × 2 table. It approximates the relative risk when the health outcome is rare:

$$OR = \frac{\frac{a}{b}}{\frac{c}{d}} = \frac{ad}{bc}$$

To see why the odds ratio approximates the relative risk when the health outcome is rare, consider an example with child injury mortality. Suppose the child injury mortality rate in one state is 34 per 100,000 children, and 26 per 100,000 children in another. For illustration, assume that each state has a child population of 100,000. Then the 2 × 2 table to compare these two mortality rates would look as follows:

Child Injury Mortality

		Yes	No	
State I	Yes	34	99,966	100,000
State II	No	26	99,974	100,000
		60	199,940	200,000

$$RR = \frac{\dfrac{34}{100,000}}{\dfrac{26}{100,000}} = \frac{34}{26} = 1.3$$

$$OR = \frac{\dfrac{34}{99,966}}{\dfrac{26}{99,974}} = \frac{34.01}{26.01} = 1.3$$

When the incidence or prevalence rate of an outcome in a population is very small, the difference between using a + b and c + d, or only b and d in the denominators is negligible. As the incidence or prevalence becomes higher, however, the difference between the two measures becomes greater with the odds ratio always being greater than the relative risk.

Suppose the data in the above example are for the number of two-year-old children receiving fewer than five well child visits so that the prevalence rates are 34 per 100 two-year-olds (34%) and 26 per 100 two-year-olds (26%) instead of 34 and 26 per 100,000:

< 5 Well Child Visits in the First Two Years of Life

		Yes	No	
State I	Yes	34,000	66,000	100,000
State II	No	26,000	74,000	100,000
		60,000	140,000	200,000

$$RR = \frac{\dfrac{34,000}{100,000}}{\dfrac{26,000}{100,000}} = \frac{34}{26} = 1.3$$

$$OR = \frac{\dfrac{34,000}{66,000}}{\dfrac{26,000}{74,000}} = \frac{51.5}{35.1} = 1.5$$

This more commonly occurring outcome yields a relative risk and odds ratio that are noticeably different. With a slightly less common occurrence such as low birthweight which, although measured per 100 births, typically ranges from 5% to 15 %, the relative risk and odds ratio will be quite close. If we were to compare low birthweight rates of 13 % and 10 %, for example, the odds ratio would be 1.34, barely larger than the relative risk of 1.3.

Because the relative risk is a comparison of two cumulative incidence rates, and the odds ratio is a comparison of two odds, the interpretation of the results is somewhat different. The relative risk is a direct comparison of probabilities so that we can say from our example with childhood injury that the children in State I have 1.3 times the risk (probability) of dying from an injury than the children in State II. On the other hand, the odds ratio is not a direct comparison of probabilities so we say that the children in State I are 1.5 times as likely to die from an injury as the children in State II. When relative prevalence is used, the comparison is between two probabilities of "having" a health status outcome.

The relative risk and relative prevalence are generally considered to be preferable to the odds ratio because they are directly related to the probability of developing or having a health outcome. The odds ratio, however, can be used when sampling strategies aimed at studying rare events yield artificial estimates of n_1 and n_2 making the RR and RP impossible to calculate. In addition, the odds ratio has become accepted as a robust measure in and of itself and is sometimes used even when it would be possible to calculate the RR and RP.

Question:

Calculate the relative risk (RR) and odds ratio (OR) using the 2 × 2 table for cocaine use during pregnancy and low birthweight:

		Low Birthweight		
		Yes	No	
Cocaine	Yes	130	370	500
Use	No	870	13,630	14,500
		1,000	14,000	15,000

Answer:

LBW among cocaine users is $130/500 \times 100$ or 26% (p_1)
LBW among non-users is $870/14,500 \times 100$ or 6% (p_2)
Overall LBW is $1,000/15,000 \times 100$ or 6.7% (p_0)

$$RR = \frac{\dfrac{130}{500}}{\dfrac{870}{14,500}} = \frac{0.26}{0.06} = 4.3$$

$$OR = \frac{\dfrac{130}{370}}{\dfrac{870}{13,630}} = \frac{0.35}{0.064} = 5.5$$

The relative risk, relative prevalence, and odds ratio can theoretically range from 0 to positive infinity, with their expected values, assuming no association, being 1. In other words, the ratio is 0 when the proportion in the numerator is 0 regardless of the value of the proportion in the denominator. The ratio can be infinitely large when the proportion in the numerator is infinitely larger than the one in the denominator. If the two proportions are equal, then the ratio of one to the other is 1.

This non-symmetric distribution, with half of the possible values lying between 0 and 1 and the other half lying between one and infinity, is not easy to evaluate using the conventional statistical tests. These ratio measures are usually transformed, therefore, using the natural logarithm to yield distributions symmetric around an expected value of 0 and approximately normal in shape, analogous to the distributions of the difference measures. For ease of interpretation and reporting, the measures and their confidence limits are transformed back to their original form after performing the desired statistical tests.

The statistical tests for the relative risk and odds ratio are as follows:

Relative Risk and Relative Prevalence

$$z = \frac{\ln\left(\frac{r_1}{r_2}\right) - 0}{\sqrt{\left(\frac{1}{a} \times \frac{b}{n_1}\right) + \left(\frac{1}{c} \times \frac{d}{n_2}\right)}}$$

Odds Ratio

$$z = \frac{\ln\left(\frac{a \times d}{b \times c}\right) - 0}{\sqrt{\frac{1}{a} + \frac{1}{b} + \frac{1}{c} + \frac{1}{d}}}$$

The observed value in the z test is now either the natural logarithm of the relative risk or odds ratio and the expected value is again 0 (the natural logarithm of 1) under the null hypothesis. Standard errors have been determined for the natural logarithm of these ratio measures of association that, as usual, take account of the number of observations that contribute to the two rates, or odds. Note that for a given 2×2 table, the z tests for ratio measures and difference measures will be very close.

The formulas for the confidence limits around the relative risk, relative prevalence, and odds ratio are as follows:

$$CI_{RR \text{ and } RP} = e^{\left(\ln\left(\frac{r_1}{r_2}\right) \pm 1.96\sqrt{\left(\frac{1}{a} \times \frac{b}{n_1}\right) + \left(\frac{1}{c} \times \frac{d}{n_2}\right)}\right)}$$

$$CI_{OR} = e^{\left(\ln\left(\frac{a \times d}{b \times c}\right) \pm 1.96\sqrt{\frac{1}{a} + \frac{1}{b} + \frac{1}{c} + \frac{1}{d}}\right)}$$

After using critical values from the standard normal curve to calculate confidence limits around the natural logarithm of the relative risk, relative prevalence, or odds ratio, the limits are exponentiated in order to transform them back onto the original scale. Remember that on their original scale, the relative risk, relative prevalence and odds ratio have expected values of 1.

Example

Remember that when we tested the difference between the hypothetical infant mortality rates of 8.0 and 6.7 per 1,000 live births in County A and County B (pages 55-56) the z statistic was 0.35 and the confidence interval around the rate difference was (−5.8-8.4). Now, let's calculate the z test and confidence interval using the relative risk for the same data:

$$z = \frac{\ln\left(\frac{8.0}{6.7}\right) - 0}{\sqrt{\left(\frac{1}{11} \times \frac{1,364}{1,375}\right) + \left(\frac{1}{6} \times \frac{894}{900}\right)}}$$

$$= \frac{0.18}{0.51}$$

$$= 0.35$$

$$CI_{RR} = e^{\left(\ln\left(\frac{8.0}{6.7}\right) \pm 1.96 \sqrt{\left(\frac{1}{11} \times \frac{1,364}{1,375}\right) + \left(\frac{1}{6} \times \frac{894}{900}\right)}\right)}$$

$$= e^{0.18 \pm 1.96 \times 0.51}$$

$$= 0.44 - 3.3$$

As before, z=0.35 and since the confidence interval of 0.44-3.3 includes the expected value of 1, the county rates are not statistically different.

When we discussed measures of association based on differences, there was no good way to determine how strong the association was based on the difference alone. With ratio measures, however, there is a direct connection between the value of the ratio itself and the strength of the association. For example, two associations may be equivalently strong, with relative risks of 1.5. One of these associations may be based on proportions of 30% and 20%, a difference of 10%. The other may be based on proportions of 9% and 6%, a difference of 3%. You can see that the difference measures do not directly show the equivalence in the strength of the two associations.

The following is a guide to assessing the strength of a ratio measure of association:

Relative Risk, Relative Prevalence, or Odds Ratio		Strength of the Association
0.83-1.00	1.0- 1.2	None
0.67-0.83	1.2- 1.5	Weak
0.33-0.67	1.5- 3.0	Moderate
0.10-0.33	3.0-10.0	Strong
< 0.01	>10.0	Approaching Infinite

Of course, appropriate confidence intervals (and p-values) will influence the interpretation of the strength of an association. Here are a few examples:

RR, RP, OR	Confidence Interval	Possible Interpretation
4.3 or 0.2	0.8-8.2 or 0.1-1.3	The estimate of association is strong, but is also very unstable since the confidence interval includes 1 and is very wide. Given the high value, though, these data provide some indication that this association may be real.
3.8 or 0.3	3.0-4.4 or 0.22-0.34	The estimate of association is strong, and is also very stable since the confidence interval does not include 1 and is quite narrow. These data provide evidence of a real association.
1.6 or 0.6	1.2-2.8 or 0.4-0.8	The estimate of association is moderate and quite stable since the confidence interval does not include 1 and is fairly narrow. These data provide evidence of a real association.
1.3 or 0.8	0.6-4.6 or 0.2-1.7	The estimate of association is weak and also very unstable since the confidence interval includes 1 and is very wide. Given the low value, these data provide no evidence that this association is real.

Question:

How would you characterize the associations between smoking and low birthweight and cocaine use and low birthweight from the hypothetical population of 15,000 live births?

RR smoking and low birthweight = 9.33 / 6.0 = 1.6 (1.4-1.8)
RR cocaine and low birthweight = 26.0 / 6.0 = 4.3 (3.7-5.1)

Answer:

The association between smoking and low birthweight is moderate; that between cocaine and low birthweight is strong. The confidence intervals are quite narrow in each case, providing evidence that the associations are real.

The Preventive Fraction

The 2 × 2 table does not always have to be organized in terms of a risk factor and adverse outcome. It can also be organized to focus on a protective effect. This may be useful in a wide variety of analyses; in particular, this configuration is useful in the context of program evaluation, where a program has been designed to have a positive impact and measuring the magnitude of this impact is desired.

The 2 × 2 table below shows the data layout for enrollment in a hypothetical program designed to reduce a hypothetical adverse outcome:

		Adverse Outcome		
		Yes	No	
Program	Yes	80	920	1,000
	No	990	8,010	9,000
		1,070	8,930	10,000

Here, the relative risk is 0.08/0.11=0.73 which is protective, that is, those enrolled in the program had less risk of developing the adverse outcome than those not in the program. The rows in the 2 × 2 table have been reversed from before, with the presumably low risk group now in the first row and the higher risk group now in the second. To make sense in this situation, the attributable risk percent must be calculated as though the table were still organized in the usual form; the high-risk group as always anchors the formula, now p_2 instead of p_1. The result is the preventive fraction and can be interpreted as a measure of program effectiveness.

For the above table:

$$\text{Preventive Fraction} = \frac{p_2 - p_1}{p_2} = 1 - \text{Relative Risk} = \frac{0.11 - 0.08}{0.11} = 0.27$$

It can be said that the program is 27 % effective in reducing the adverse outcome.

Question:

Calculate the preventive fraction for the following data on infant car seat use and motor vehicle injury

		Injury		
		Yes	No	
Car Seat Use	Yes	20	4,980	5,000
	No	50	4,950	5,000
		70	9,930	10,000

Answer:

Injury rate among infants in car seats is 20/5,000 = 0.004
Injury rate among infants not in car seats is 50/5,000 = 0.01
RR = 0.004/0.01 = 0.4
1-RR, or the preventive fraction is 1-0.4 = 0.60

Using car seats for infants is 60 % effective in preventing motor vehicle injury.

ECOLOGIC ANALYSIS

The examples in the last section used the 2 × 2 table to examine the association between a risk factor and an outcome and between geographic areas and an outcome, in each case using individual level data. In other words, the smoking status of each pregnant woman, the county of residence for each pregnant woman, as well as the birthweight for each infant was known, and the state of residence and the number of well child visits for each child was known. The sample size (N) in each of the 2 × 2 tables for these examples equaled the total number of individuals for whom there was data.

Sometimes, however, an association is to be evaluated at the aggregate level and then the N in the 2 × 2 table equals the total number of *groups* observed. The groups, or units of analysis, may be geographic areas or health facilities. For instance, the smoking and low birthweight data might look like the following for 50 hypothetical counties:

	Low Birthweight		
	> 5 %*	<=5 %	
>= 20 % Smokers	25	5	30
< 20% Smokers	10	10	20
	35	15	50 counties

*5% is the Year 2000 Objective

Now, the prevalence of smoking among pregnant women in a county is the risk factor and the outcome is prevalence of low birthweight in a county. Consider some of the familiar statistics and measures of association, and the possible interpretation in this context:

$$p_1 = \frac{25}{30} = 0.83$$

$$p_2 = \frac{10}{20} = 0.50$$

$$\text{Outcome Prevalence} : p_0 = \frac{35}{50} = 0.70$$

$$\text{"Exposure" Prevalence} : \frac{30}{50} = 0.60$$

$$\text{Relative Risk} : \frac{0.83}{0.50} = 1.7$$

$$\text{Population Attributable Risk\%} : \frac{0.70 - 0.50}{0.70} \times 100 = 29\%$$

Counties with a high prevalence of smoking among pregnant women have 1.7 times the risk of not meeting the Year 2000 Objective for low birthweight. The PAR% of 29%, means that the number of counties that might meet the Year 2000 Objective if smoking prevalence could be decreased to < 20% in all of the counties would be $0.29 \times 35 \cong 10$. In other words, only 25 rather than 35 of the 50 counties would fall short of the Objective.

Historically, epidemiologists have questioned the value of ecologic analysis, since the connection between the exposure and outcome is not linked at the individual level. In other words, in the above example, it is unknown whether the women who smoked during their pregnancies are the same ones who delivered low birthweight infants.

Example

The statistical test with county as the unit of analysis is:

$$z = \frac{0.83 - 0.50}{\sqrt{0.70(1-0.70)\left(\frac{1}{30} + \frac{1}{20}\right)}} = 2.5, \quad z = \frac{\ln\left(\frac{0.83}{0.50}\right)}{\sqrt{\left(\frac{1}{25} \times \frac{5}{30}\right) + \left(\frac{1}{10} \times \frac{10}{20}\right)}} = 2.1, \quad z = \frac{\ln\left(\frac{25 \times 10}{5 \times 10}\right)}{\sqrt{\frac{1}{25} + \frac{1}{5} + \frac{1}{10} + \frac{1}{10}}} = 2.4$$

Difference   Relative Risk   Odds Ratio

Whichever test is used, the z value is greater than the usual critical value of 1.96, so the p-value is less than 0.05. The tests indicate that higher prevalence of smoking among pregnant women in a county is associated with higher prevalence of low birthweight.

Categorizing the county prevalence rates of smoking at < 20 % and >= 20% and the rates of low birthweight at <= 5 % and > 5% illustrates the importance of choosing appropriate breakpoints for continuous variables that are transformed to fit into the framework of the 2 × 2 table. This is true for individual level data as well, when the exposure is not simply present or absent but has many values that are converted to a dichotomous form. If the categories are not chosen appropriately, misclassification has in effect occurred, and the results of the risk measures may be biased.

FINAL NOTES ON INTERPRETING 2 X 2 TABLES

We have seen that ratio measures and difference measures derived from a 2 × 2 table provide different types of information. The relative risk and odds ratio are used to measure the strength or the magnitude of an association between an exposure or risk factor, and a health outcome; the attributable risk measures are used to gauge the potential public health impact of an exposure.

In addition, the interpretation of the epidemiologic measures of risk must take into account the structure and type of data being used. Just as the assumption of causality did not hold when county was the exposure variable, so too this assumption may be questioned when data are at the aggregate level or when the data are for service or systems variables. Since the traditional epidemiologic risk measures are used with many kinds of data, however, terminology and assumptions may have to be modified to accommodate a broader public health interpretation.

In any case, the 2 × 2 table remains a very useful tool for organizing data whether or not particular risk measures will be reported. It helps the analyst clarify the questions of interest, permits exploration of the impact of different categorization schemes, and provides a format for exploration of hypothetical changes in health status, health services, or health systems.

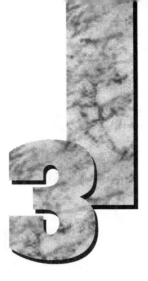

Analytic Epidemiology and Multivariable Methods

by Deborah Rosenberg, PhD and Arden Handler, DrPH

Multivariable methods are a tool for characterizing the complex relationships among individual, medical and social factors which define the context of maternal and child health. When using these methods, a clear conceptual framework should drive both the study design and the data analysis. Deciding which study type is appropriate, which, if any, multivariable model is appropriate, which variables will be included, the definitions of these variables, and the coding for each, is a prerequisite for meaningful epidemiologic analysis.

RESEARCH DESIGNS IN ANALYTIC EPIDEMIOLOGY

Up to this point, all of the examples of measures of association and hypothesis testing have assumed that complete population data, or data from a random sample are available. Sometimes, however, these types of data are not available, or it is not feasible or efficient to use them in this form. Sometimes, in order to investigate a particular question, more complex research designs are required. Sometimes, although the data you are using are from a random sample or are population based, it is important to impose a design structure as a way to help with decisions about the appropriate measures of association to investigate and report.

The research designs that generate the types of data that can be categorized in 2 × 2 tables are derived from analytic epidemiology (the study of the determinants and risk of disease) as opposed to descriptive epidemiology, which is the study of the patterns and frequency of disease. These analytic study designs are often called *observational* because they were developed to examine associations between risk factors and outcomes, in contrast to *intervention* studies that explore the associations between interventions and outcomes, and in epidemiology are called experimental studies or clinical trials.

The two designs that are considered the workhorse designs of analytic epidemiology are the *cohort study (exposure → disease)* and the *case-control study (disease → exposure)*. We will discuss these as well as those designs that are based on data from the entire population *(disease ↔ exposure)* and those based on ecologic comparisons. These latter two study types are typically not considered as strong as either the cohort or case-control designs, but they are commonly used in the public health setting. Our goal is not to provide an in-depth review of epidemiologic study designs but rather to provide some relevant basic points about each design type. We refer the reader to Hennekens and Buring, *Epidemiology in Medicine* and Rothman, *Modern Epidemiology* for more details on these study designs.

Cohort Study

This study design is considered the gold standard when exploring the association between a risk factor or participation in a health program, and health status outcomes or health events. When data are collected on a population that is free of disease, it is possible to follow the cohorts of exposed and unexposed individuals from exposure to outcome, and the incidence of the outcome in both the exposed and unexposed groups can be generated. The ratio of these two risks is the relative risk as described in the previous module.

**Cohort Design I: Sampling from a Disease-Free Population
Prior to Knowing Exposure Status**

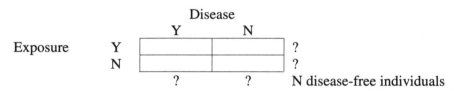

This cohort design is based on sampling only individuals who do not have the outcome of interest at the beginning of the study. The number of individuals in the four cells of the table, therefore, is unknown until the end of the study at which time the calculation of disease incidence as well as of exposure prevalence is possible. This study design is, by definition, prospective.

Sometimes, if an exposure of interest is quite rare, sampling is carried out separately among those with and without the exposure in order to insure adequate numbers of exposed individuals.

**Cohort Design II: Sampling from a Disease-Free Population
According to Exposure Status (n_1 and n_2)**

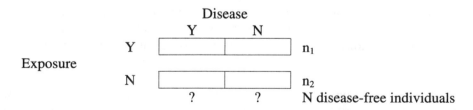

Although the numbers of exposed and unexposed are fixed, the number of individuals in the four cells of the table is still unknown until the end of the study at which time calculation of disease incidence is possible. The prevalence of exposure, however, cannot be estimated since n_1 and n_2 have been fixed by the sampling design. This design is also, by definition, prospective.

While the cohort study is considered optimal, it is expensive and time consuming to follow a cohort of individuals forward in time to examine differential experiences or outcomes. For instance, to assess the effect of smoking on tubal pregnancy, large numbers of women would need to be followed for multiple years, a task which is usually beyond the resource capabilities of professionals in state and local health agencies.

Case-Control Study

The case-control study is more commonly used than the cohort study because it is less expensive to accumulate cases of an outcome of interest and subsequently gather controls who are similar enough to the cases to allow for a comparison of differential exposure. Case-control studies are mounted when the outcome of interest is very rare, and drawing a random sample of cases from the population would therefore yield too few cases over too long a time period and would involve too much expense. While we often use the terms cases and controls, a true case control study involves a retrospective assessment of differential exposure between the two comparison groups.

The Case Control Design: Sampling from m_1 and m_2

		Disease			
		Yes	No		
Exposure	Yes	a	b	n_1	
	No	c	d	n_2	
		m_1	m_2	N individuals	

In a case control study, sampling is carried out separately among those with and without the outcome in order to insure adequate numbers of diseased individuals. The numbers in all four cells of the table can be filled in at the time of data collection. Here, calculation of disease incidence is not possible since m_1 and m_2 have been fixed by the sampling design. The prevalence of exposure, however, can be estimated.

Because disease incidence cannot be calculated in a case control study, the relative risk cannot be used as a measure of association. Instead, the measure of association between exposure and outcome, the odds ratio (ad/bc), as described in the previous module, is used as an approximation of the relative risk. For instance, if 100 children with asthma and 100 children without asthma were sampled in order to examine the relationship between exposure to cockroaches and occurrence of asthma, the incidence of asthma among the exposed and unexposed could not be generated since the sampling design has created a distorted distribution of individuals such that the overall incidence of disease falsely appears to be 50% .

Sometimes, case-control studies are mounted within a cohort study in which individuals have been followed over time and for whom information has been collected on a variety of outcomes. One can use all of the cases of the outcome of interest found in this cohort and take a sample from the remaining individuals to serve as the controls and then examine the exposure-outcome relationship in the combined group. Because the cases are generated from within a cohort study, this is called a *nested case-control study*.

Data from the Entire Population

In state and local health agencies data are typically available on the entire population, those with and without disease and those with and without exposure. These data are usually thought of as cross-sectional since collection or sampling of the exposure and outcome information is at the same point in time.

Usually, data collected or sampled in this fashion are considered prevalence data and the relationship between an exposure and an outcome can be considered the ratio of two prevalence rates, or relative prevalence.

Cross-sectional Design: Sampling from the Entire Population

		Disease		
		Yes	No	
Exposure	Yes	a	b	n_1
	No	c	d	n_2
		m_1	m_2	N individuals

In a cross-sectional design, individuals from the entire relevant population are sampled, including those with and without the outcome of interest. The numbers in all four cells of the table can be filled in at the time of data collection and the distribution of individuals is not distorted by the sampling design.

With cross-sectional data, when the outcome is clearly new cases (e.g., low birthweight or asthma deaths), occurrence of the outcome can actually be considered incidence and the ratio of these two incidence rates is the relative risk. Moreover, when information about the timing or biological sequence of events (e.g., smoking and low birthweight) is known, it is possible to make inferences about causality. Sometimes, cross-sectional data collected on a group of individuals over time, are used to retrospectively construct a cohort of exposed and unexposed individuals. This retrospective cohort study is manageable and efficient, but depends upon reliable documentation of both exposure and outcome in the data-set of interest.

Ecologic Designs

We can also generate 2×2 tables from data in which our exposure and outcome cannot be linked at the individual level. For example, the smoking and low birthweight data for 50 counties described in Module 2 is an example of data drawn from an ecologic study. While the association between two data elements that are not linked at the individual level is considered a cause for concern with respect to making assumptions about individuals (*ecologic fallacy*), more current thinking holds that the ecologic level of analysis may be an appropriate and valid tool in its own right. While we usually focus on individual risk factors and outcomes, examination of the relationship between population risk factors or exposure to a program on a population level, and population outcomes is also of value as we develop population based intervention strategies.

Ecologic Design: Data are not Linked at the Individual Level

		Disease %		
		High	Low	
Exposure %	High	a	b	n_1
	Low	c	d	n_2
		m_1	m_2	N groups

In an ecologic design, the data for exposure and disease are used in aggregated form and cannot be linked at the individual level. The fours cells of the table, therefore, do not contain the number of individuals with a given joint exposure-outcome status, but rather contain the number of groups (usually geographic areas or health facilities) with a given joint exposure-outcome status.

DESIGNS FOR PROGRAM EVALUATION

While analytic epidemiologic designs have been the focus of this module, when an MCH professional in a state or local health agency confronts the questions that need to be answered to improve programming on behalf of women, children and families, there are actually a multitude of study designs from which to choose. In particular, one needs to consider whether the designs which are drawn from the social sciences or clinical research, called experimental and quasi-experimental designs, are appropriate, or whether the epidemiologic analytic designs described above are more relevant. To make this decision, one needs to understand the basic distinction between these different types of designs and to examine the appropriateness of the design type for the question at hand. Clearly, we can approach study design from many vantage points but our aim, no matter what our strategy, is to develop a design which is as free from bias as feasible given the constraints of resources and time, as well as ethical and political realities.

Choosing a Study Design

In general, study designs that focus on determining if there is a causal relationship between exposures and outcomes have traditionally been divided into two groups:

1. **Intervention studies**: designs in which the exposure is *manipulated* by the investigator/public health professional. These designs come from a variety of fields including clinical medicine, epidemiology and the social sciences. As mentioned above, intervention studies in the field of epidemiology and clinical medicine are often called clinical trials, while in the social sciences they are often called experimental designs (with random assignment to groups) or quasi-experimental designs (without random assignment to groups).

2. **Observational studies**: designs in which the exposure *is not manipulated* by the investigator/public health professional. These designs come from the field of *analytic epidemiology* and were initially developed for situations in which the exposures of interest are observed phenomena, as opposed to interventions or programs. The major designs in this category are the cohort and case-control study designs described above.

Historically, observational designs were reserved exclusively for examining risk factors and outcomes. However, as epidemiologists have become more active in health services research and in conducting program evaluations, they have begun to use observational designs to examine the relationship between participation in programs and health status outcomes. When evaluating programs, however, there has been de facto *manipulation* of the exposure, not just *observation* of the exposure. The manipulation may have been at the policy level, not directly controlled by the evaluator, but manipulation has occurred nonetheless. Therefore, manipulation of the exposure no longer defines the difference between intervention and observational studies. When the exposure is a health program or policy, then, what influences whether the study design is drawn from the realm of observational studies (cohort and case-control studies) or from the realm of intervention studies (quasi-experimental and experimental designs)?

When the exposure is a health program or policy, the choice of using observational designs instead of quasi-experimental/experimental designs is dependent on whether there is the theoretical possibility of collecting pretest or baseline data from the same units (e.g., individuals, clinics, provider practices) on which there is an outcome measurement:

- In observational studies there are two phenomena of interest, an exposure which can be a program or policy, and an outcome, such as health status or use of health services.

- In experimental and quasi-experimental designs there are also two phenomena of interest, an exposure and an outcome, but the outcome *can be measured at two points* in time, pretest/baseline data (whether one collects it or not) and posttest data (whether one collects it or not.)

In program evaluation, experimental designs and quasi-experimental designs are usually used when there is outcome information at baseline about one or more groups, an intervention takes place, and outcome information can also be collected on the same group or groups subsequent to the intervention. The research question can be stated as, "does the intervention *change* the outcome status of the individuals being studied?" Observational designs are used in program evaluation when an intervention takes place, outcome information is subsequently collected, but there was no theoretical possibility to collect outcome information at baseline on the same units or subjects because the outcome can only occur following the exposure (i.e., many health status outcomes). Now, the research question is stated as, "does the intervention have an impact on *whether* the outcome occurs?"

Observational designs can be thought of as analogous to post-test-only designs in the experimental/quasi-experimental design framework. Posttest only designs, however, particularly those without random assignment, are considered some of the weaker designs of this paradigm since they cannot control for differences in outcome status prior to the intervention. When a health outcome can occur only once, however, in effect there are no baseline differences to account for; all individuals in the study have the same status prior to the intervention. In this context, concern about the weakness of the posttest only, or observational design, is unwarranted.

Comment

Experimental designs involve a program or a treatment, an outcome measure, and a comparison from which change due to the program or treatment can be inferred. Experimental designs involve random assignment to a "treatment" or control group.

Random assignment is the use of a process of random selection as to who receives the treatment and who does not receive the treatment under study. Random assignment creates theoretically equivalent comparison groups.

Quasi-experimental designs involve a program or treatment and an outcome measure but the comparison groups from which change is to be inferred are not created through random assignment. The comparison groups are nonequivalent so attributing cause to the program or treatment is more difficult than in an experimental design.

For more information on experimental designs refer to Campbell and Stanley's *Experimental and Quasi-Experimental Designs for Research on Teaching*; for more information on quasi-experimental designs refer to Cook and Campbell's *Quasi-Experimentation: Design and Analysis Issues for Field Settings*.

Example One. WIC participants in one county are participating in a variety of interventions to change behaviors; two of interest to a local health agency are a household budgeting workshop and a breastfeeding workshop. The local health agency is interested in the effect of these workshops on client behavior.

To study the effect of a household budgeting workshop on the purchasing behavior of WIC participants, the program evaluator is likely to choose an experimental or quasi-experimental design because the collection of pretest data (purchasing behavior) on the same subjects before and after the workshop is theoretically possible.

However, if the evaluator is interested in the impact of a WIC breastfeeding workshop provided during pregnancy on the breastfeeding behavior of first-time mothers, then the evaluator is likely to choose an observational study design. Since the population has yet to experience the behavior in the particular episode under study, there is no theoretical possibility of administering a pretest to the actual participants in the intervention. In other words, primiparous mothers do not have prior breastfeeding behavior, so it is not possible to obtain baseline data. Instead, an epidemiologic cohort study design, in which those exposed to the workshop and those not exposed to the workshop are followed to observe breastfeeding behavior, can be employed.

In both of the above scenarios, the exposure has been manipulated. However, in the first scenario there is the theoretical possibility of collecting pretest data on the individuals in the workshop and therefore an experimental or quasi-experimental design is selected. In the second scenario there is no possibility of collecting pretest data on these individuals so an observational design is chosen.

Example Two. The state health agency is interested in evaluating the impact of a teenage pregnancy prevention program on the *knowledge, attitudes and sexual practices* of not previously pregnant high-risk adolescent females engaged in sexual activity which places them at risk of STDS/HIV and/or pregnancy. There is also an interest in exploring the impact of this program on pregnancy rates. The program has been implemented in several counties and is limited to 50 female teens per site; those who are eligible for the program but are unable to participate due to space limitations are placed on a waiting list (there is no random assignment). In order to examine the impact of the program on participants' knowledge, attitudes and sexual behavior, information on these three domains can be collected before the teens begin the program and then again at one or more points after their participation in the program is ended. Information on pregnancy can be obtained through follow-up for several years after participation in the program is concluded.

If the program manager/evaluator chooses to collect pre-test and post-test information on knowledge, attitudes and behavior from program participants and the individuals on the waiting list, the design would be quasi-experimental. When considering the relationship between exposure to the intervention and the occurrence of pregnancy, on the other hand, the evaluator is likely to conduct an epidemiologic cohort study because the event of pregnancy can only occur after (during) the intervention.

Use of Historical or Community Controls

For many program evaluations in which the outcomes are such that baseline or pre-test data on the outcome of interest cannot be collected on the unique individuals who have participated in the intervention, the evaluator can often obtain an indirect pretest measure from historical or community controls. For example, in the study described above of breastfeeding behavior, historical data on the breastfeeding behavior of first time mothers in the WIC program might be compared to the breastfeeding behavior of workshop participants and non-participants.

Likewise, in the study described above of pregnancy prevention among high risk teens the evaluator might also examine the pregnancy rates of high risk teens in the communities in which the intervention took place before its implementation and compare these to the rates for the teen participants and non-participants in the program. In both of these cases, the evaluator is establishing a baseline from community or population data rather than from the identified participants or non-participants in the program.

Summary

In sum, when the goal is to answer questions about programs, the more useful distinction between observational studies and quasi-experimental and experimental designs is not manipulation of exposure but rather whether there is the theoretical possibility of obtaining pre-test or baseline measures on *the same units or subjects* for which there is outcome measurement. Selecting the type of study design from one paradigm or another is dependent on the question being asked, the kinds of data available, whether baseline information is theoretically possible, and the resources that can be brought to bear on the task.

While naming the study design is less important than developing a design that can answer the questions of interest, choosing nomenclature helps one to think through the appropriate measures of association, the relevant statistical tests, and the biases that may affect whether it will be possible to establish that an association between a program or policy and an outcome is in fact genuine.

Question:

Which study design would you choose for the following? Which is the exposure and which is the outcome?

1. The state health agency is exploring a variety of strategies to increase immunization rates of pediatric providers. Pediatric providers are randomly assigned to one of three interventions. The outcome of interest is immunization rates of two-year-olds.

2. The state health agency is examining the impact of participation in primary care case-management for children with special health care needs on reduction in the use of hospital emergency rooms for primary care visits. Children are assigned to primary care case-management on a first-come first served basis; those on the waiting list constitute the comparison group.

3. The state health agency has designed an asthma prevention program for a cohort of low birthweight infants who had respiratory problems at birth; only LBW infants at three hospitals in the state have been selected for participation. The goal is to follow those exposed to the intervention and those not exposed to the intervention to determine the incidence rate of asthma through age five.

Answer:

1. The evaluator would logically choose an experimental design. Providers are the units that are randomly assigned to treatment, and immunization rates for two-year-olds in each provider's practice can be measured before and after the implementation of the intervention.

2. The evaluator would logically choose a quasi-experimental design as emergency room use before and after the intervention can be examined, and a non-equivalent comparison group is available.

3. The evaluator would logically choose a cohort study design following the exposed and unexposed infants to examine the difference in incidence rates of asthma between the two groups. There is no possibility of a pre-test or baseline measure for this group of infants.

ADJUSTMENT FOR CONFOUNDING

How do we know if an association between a risk factor / program / system change and a health event / program / system outcome is real?

We have described the use of statistical testing to evaluate whether an association is due to chance or reflects a "true" relationship. While we may discover statistically significant results, statistical significance is only one part of the picture. The relationship between the two variables may actually be due to bias in the design of the study or to confounding of the relationship between the two variables by a third variable. We have discussed the two major types of bias, information bias and selection bias, previously. To discover bias that might distort the relationship between an exposure and outcome, it is essential to use critical thinking skills to judge whether differences between groups are the result of disparities in the way the groups were selected or are the result of differential ascertainment of information on both exposures and outcomes for the groups.

Sometimes even when the study design is free of bias, an apparent association may not be "real" but may instead be due to the mixing of a third factor with the exposure and the outcome. For example, if one finds a relationship between participation in the WIC program and increased birthweight of infants, it is necessary to consider whether a third factor such as age of the WIC participants, parity of the WIC participants, or health behaviors of the WIC participants may explain the relationship between WIC and increased infant birthweight. Confounding, unlike bias, cannot be eliminated by improving the study design; confounding is a reflection of the complex interrelationship between variables in the real world.

To be eligible as a confounder, a third factor or variable must meet the following criteria:

1. It must be a risk factor for the outcome, independent of its association with the risk factor or exposure under study. It does not have to be causally associated with the outcome, but simply correlated with it.
2. It must be correlated with the risk factor or exposure under study, independent of its association with the outcome.
3. It must not be in the hypothesized causal pathway *between* the risk factor and outcome.

EVALUATING THE ROLE OF CONFOUNDING

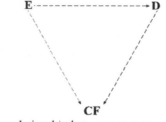

Interrelationship between an exposure (E),
confounding factor (?CF), and disease (D).

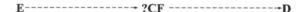

Interrelationship between an exposure (E), disease (D),
and a potential confounding factor (?CF) which is in
the causal pathway and thus *not* a confounder.

From Epidemiology in Medicine, Charles Hennekens and Julie Buring. Copyright © 1988 by Little, Brown & Company. Used by permission of Little, Brown & Company.

How do we assess whether a third factor is a confounder of the association of interest?

When evaluating confounding, person variables such as ethnicity/race, age, parity, education, health insurance status and socioeconomic status are typically the "usual suspects". It is also desirable to consider other variables as potential confounders as well; this decision should be based on both what is available in the data-set at hand and what is known about the relationship under consideration.

Steps in Evaluating Confounding Based on Analysis of 2×2 Tables

The following steps are those typically used when your measure of association is the odds ratio or relative risk. The aim is to determine if the crude OR or RR is different than the odds ratio or relative risk obtained after adjustment for a third variable. Determining whether a difference between the crude and adjusted measures is meaningful is a matter of judgement since there is no formal test for the presence of confounding.

First, explore whether the third factor is related to the two variables of interest. If it is not related to both variables, it cannot be a confounder.

Second, if the third factor is related to the two variables of interest, conduct stratified analysis. To conduct stratified analysis using 2×2 tables, the exposure and the outcome variables must be dichotomous, and the potential confounder must be categorical although not necessarily dichotomous. In stratified analysis, one examines several two by two tables; each table shows the relationship between the two variables of interest at each level of the third variable.

Third, compare the crude odds ratio or crude relative risk to the weighted average of the stratum specific odds ratios or relative risks generated from stratified analysis. These stratum specific measures are unconfounded estimates of the relationship between the two variables at each level of the third variable. If the weighted odds ratio or relative risk is different than the crude (unstratified) estimate of association, then confounding is present.

The formulas for the weighted (adjusted) estimates are extensions of the formulas for the crude relative risk and odds ratio. The numerator of the adjusted relative risk is a weighted sum of the numerators of the relative risk in each stratum; the denominator is a weighted sum of the denominators of the relative risk in each stratum. Likewise, the numerator of the adjusted odds ratio is a weighted sum of the numerators of the odds ratio in each stratum; the denominator is a weighted sum of the denominators of the odds ratio in each stratum. In both measures, the weights are based on the total sample size.

Rothman - Boice Summary Relative Risk :

$$= \frac{\sum\limits_{i=1}^{\#\text{strata}} \frac{a_i n_{2i}}{N_i}}{\sum\limits_{i=1}^{\#\text{strata}} \frac{c_i n_{1i}}{N_i}}$$

Mantel - Haenszel Summary Odds Ratio :

$$= \frac{\displaystyle\sum_{i=1}^{\#\,\text{strata}} \frac{a_i d_i}{N_i}}{\displaystyle\sum_{i=1}^{\#\,\text{strata}} \frac{b_i c_i}{N_i}}$$

The confidence limits for the adjusted relative risk and odds ratio are likewise extensions of the formulas for their unadjusted counterparts. They are based on a weighted sum of the standard errors of the stratum specific estimates. Statistical and epidemiologic software will calculate the appropriate confidence intervals for adjusted measures.

Evaluating Effect Modification Based on Analysis of 2×2 Tables

Stratified analysis can also be used to identify whether a third factor is an effect modifier of the relationship between a risk factor and an outcome. While a confounder uniformly (or close to uniformly) changes the association between the exposure and outcome across all strata of the third variable, an effect modifier differentially changes the association between the exposure and outcome across the strata. Also called interaction, effect modification is present if the relationship between the risk factor and the outcome is different, either in direction or magnitude, at each level of the third factor. The focus when assessing effect modification, then, is on comparing the relative risks or odds ratios from stratum to stratum rather than on comparing the crude and the weighted summary estimate which is appropriate for assessing confounding.

A test statistic, the *Breslow-Day Test for Homogeneity of the Odds Ratio* can be used to statistically determine if effect modification is present. However, it is best to use this test in conjunction with a non-statistical assessment of the stratum specific estimates incorporating what is known about the sample size in each stratum. If effect modification is present, the weighted summary measure should not be used; the stratum specific estimates should be used instead.

In the presence of confounding an adjusted measure appropriately controls for a third factor and it is unnecessary to focus on the third factor itself. In contrast, in the presence of effect modification, the third factor is critical to understanding the differential impact that the risk factor, program, or systems measure is having on the outcome of interest.

Suppose the following 2×2 table illustrates the crude association between a hypothetical "exposure" and outcome. The crude relative risk is 1.67, indicating a moderate association.

Crude Association

Outcome

		Y	N	
E X P	Y	500	4,000	4,500
	N	700	9,800	10,500
		1,200	13,800	15,000

$$\text{Crude RR} = \frac{11.11}{6.67} = 1.67$$

Next, to investigate possible confounding or effect modification, the data are stratified according to levels of a third factor. The association between the hypothetical exposure and outcome is presented below under three conditions: no confounding, confounding, and effect modification. In all three sets of 2×2 tables, the strata can be re-combined to yield the crude table as shown above. For this example, the third factor has two levels resulting in two strata, although a third factor may have any number of levels resulting in the equivalent number of strata.

No Confounding or Effect Modification

Stratum 1
Outcome

		Y	N	
E X P	Y	250	1,250	1,500
	N	350	3,150	3,500
		600	4,400	5,000

Stratum 2
Outcome

		Y	N	
E X P	Y	250	2,750	3,000
	N	350	6,650	7,000
		600	9,400	10,000

$$RR_1 = \frac{16.67}{10.00} = 1.67$$

$$RR_2 = \frac{8.33}{5.00} = 1.67$$

$$\text{Adj. RR} = 1.67$$

Confounding

Stratum 1
Outcome

		Y	N	
E X P	Y	350	2,150	2,500
	N	250	2,250	2,500
		600	4,400	5,000

Stratum 2
Outcome

		Y	N	
E X P	Y	150	1,850	2,000
	N	450	7,550	8,000
		600	9,400	10,000

$$RR_1 = \frac{14.0}{10.0} = 1.40$$

$$RR_2 = \frac{7.50}{5.63} = 1.33$$

$$\text{Adj. RR} = 1.37$$

Effect Modification

Stratum 1
Outcome

		Y	N	
E X P	Y	365	2,135	2,500
	N	175	2,325	2,500
		540	4,460	5,000

Stratum 2
Outcome

		Y	N	
E X P	Y	135	1,865	2,000
	N	525	7,475	8,000
		660	9,340	10,000

$$RR_1 = \frac{14.6}{7.00} = 2.09$$

$$RR_2 = \frac{6.75}{6.56} = 1.03$$

In the leftmost set of tables, there is no confounding by the third factor since the adjusted relative risk of 1.67 is exactly the same as the crude relative risk seen above (1.67). In the middle set of tables, the third factor would typically be considered a confounder since the adjusted relative risk of 1.37 is quite different from the crude relative risk, and this average mirrors fairly well the relative risks in each stratum. In the rightmost set of tables, the third factor would typically be considered an effect modifier since the relative risks of 2.1 and 1.03 in each stratum are very different from each other, and in fact the Breslow-Day Test for Homogeneity of the Odds Ratios shows them to be significantly different from each other ($p=0.001$). Although an adjusted relative risk could also be calculated here, resulting in a value of 1.51, this average does not mirror the relative risks in each stratum and should not be used.

Notice that lack of confounding does not necessarily mean that the two strata are identical. Looking again at the leftmost set of tables, the outcome rates of 16.67 and 10.00 among the exposed and unexposed respectively in the first stratum are each higher than the outcome rates of 8.33 and 5.00 among the analogous groups in the second stratum, even though they result in the same relative risks. This is because the third factor is related to the outcome, with overall rates of 12% (600/5,000) and 6% (600/10,000) in the two strata, compared to the crude rate of 8% (1,200/15,000). No confounding exists, however, because the third factor is not related to the exposure since 30% of the individuals in each stratum are exposed (1,500/5,000 and 3,000/10,000), exactly the same percentage as in the crude table (4,500/15,000). Remember that confounding does not exist if a third factor is unrelated to both exposure and outcome, or if it is related to one or the other, but not to both.

When confounding does exist, it may be because the third factor is positively correlated with both the exposure and outcome, because it is negatively correlated with both the exposure and outcome, or because it is positively correlated with either the exposure or outcome and negatively correlated with the other. Looking again at the middle set of tables, in addition to the third factor being related to the outcome with the overall rates of 12% and 6% in the two strata, it is now also related to the exposure with 50% (2,500/5,000) and 20% (2,000/10,000) being exposed in the two strata compared with the 30% (4,500/15,000) in the crude table. Here, the third factor is positively correlated with both exposure and outcome; both the prevalence of exposure and the incidence of the outcome are higher in the first stratum.

Question:

Using the following information , determine whether there is confounding or effect modification present. Assume a narrow confidence band around each relative risk.

	Crude	Adjusted	Stratum 1	Stratum 2	Confounding?	Effect Modification?
1.	1.8	1.8	1.7	1.9		
2.	1.8	1.5	0.9	2.5		
3.	1.8	1.4	1.4	1.5		
4.	1.8	1.8	3.2	1.0		
5.	0.5	0.6	0.5	0.7		

Answer:

	Crude	Adjusted	Stratum 1	Stratum 2	Confounding?	Effect Modification?
1.	1.8	1.8	1.7	1.9	N	N
2.	1.8	1.5	0.9	2.5	NA	Y
3.	1.8	1.4	1.4	1.5	Y	N
4.	1.8	1.8	3.2	1.0	NA	Y
5.	0.5	0.6	0.5	0.6	Y	N

Note that once the presence of effect modification is identified, as in #2 and #4 above, the concept of confounding is not applicable. Also, if confidence limits had not been assumed to be narrow, but instead were wide due to small sample size, the apparent effect modification in #2 and #4 might not be real. The stability of estimates, in this case relative risks, must be considered when assessing both potential confounding and effect modification.

In addition, care must be taken when assessing differences in estimates with values < 1. For example, the crude and adjusted estimates of 0.5 and 0.6 in #5 do not appear very different, but remember that the relative risk can range from 0 to infinity and that half of all possible values are < 1. If the values of 0.5 and 0.6 are inverted ($1/0.5=2.0$ and $1/0.6=1.67$), then the difference between them is more readily seen.

Typically, in the analysis of the relationship between an exposure and an outcome, multiple confounders are considered. The analyst is encouraged to examine the relationship of each potential confounder with the association under interest separately before proceeding to consider the joint effects of many potential confounders using multivariable methods. Once multiple confounders or effect modifiers are identified, multivariable methods can be used to obtain the best estimate of the association between the exposure and the outcome of interest. Stratified analysis may be used to simultaneously adjust for two or more factors, but very quickly this type of analysis becomes inefficient. Regression approaches are better suited for this situation and will be discussed later in this module.

CONFOUNDING AND STANDARDIZATION OF RATES

In the previous section, we discussed the concepts of confounding and effect modification. In analytic epidemiology, when the purpose is to investigate a potentially etiologic, or causal, association between a risk factor and an outcome, "controlling for" confounding is an essential step in obtaining an unbiased estimate of the strength of the hypothesized relationship. In a public health context, when the purpose is to compare health status in different populations—when membership in a population is the "exposure"—standardization of rates is often carried out in an effort to insure that the comparison is made accounting for differences in fundamental, structural characteristics. In either case, the goal is to account for any mixing of a third factor (or multiple other factors) with the primary association of interest.

Several terms, then, are used to describe methods that address potential confounding. Each term is typically applied in a particular analytic context, but the goal of accounting for confounding factors is the same.

"Standardization"
"Adjustment"
"Controlling for"
"Stratified Analysis"

As we've already seen, the process of accounting for confounding involves separating the data into a series of strata and then applying a method that yields a summary or average estimate, weighted by the distribution of observations across the strata.

Standardization of rates has been most commonly used in epidemiology when comparing the mortality experience across populations. Typically, the comparisons are between large populations, often between nations, or sometimes between states. The objective is to adjust for societal level features that fundamentally distinguish the populations being compared. The age structure of a population, for instance, is a marker of social, economic, and political development in the broadest sense. Following is a series of age categories that might be used to produce an age-standardized mortality rate:

$$< 1$$
$$1\text{-}4$$
$$5\text{-}14$$
$$15\text{-}24$$
$$25\text{-}44$$
$$45\text{-}64$$
$$65\text{-}84$$
$$> 85$$

Since chronological age is positively correlated with most chronic diseases and since populations often have differing age structures, age meets the definition of a confounder and age standardized (or age-adjusted) rates are generated in order to make comparisons. For example, rates of coronary heart disease are known to increase with age. If a comparison is to be made between two geographic areas, one with 12% of its population over the age of 65, the other with only 6% of its population over the age of 65, higher death rates from CHD would be expected in the first population on the basis of this age difference alone. From a public health perspective, it is much more relevant to know if there is a difference in death rates in the two areas due to factors beyond the aging process itself—factors that may be amenable to public health interventions.

What typically distinguishes standardization of rates from other stratified methods for control of confounding is its use of an external standard. In other words, in addition to having data on the populations of interest, data from another population is used as a common benchmark. For example, the World Population, or the U.S. population from the 1940 Census, or from the 1970 Census might be used to compare U.S. and Canadian mortality rates in 1990. Sometimes an external standard may include the populations being compared, as when state rates are standardized according to national data.

In order to illustrate the process of rate standardization with an external standard, let's consider the following example comparing neonatal mortality rates in two hypothetical hospital groups in a region: one group is comprised of tertiary care hospitals with neonatal intensive care units (NICUs), the other is comprised of community hospitals which appropriately transfer the majority of high risk pregnant women for delivery at a tertiary center. The birthweight distribution in the two groups is considered a potential confounder since the tertiary care hospitals by definition serve higher risk pregnant women than do the community hospitals and birthweight is also known to be the major predictor of neonatal mortality. All live births in the state will be used as the external standard.

The data are as follows:

1. Hospital Group A: Community Hospitals

Birthweight Strata	Deaths	Births	% of Total	Stratum Specific Rate per 1000	Crude Rate per 1000
< 1500	53	150	1	353.3	
1500 – 2499	12	750	5	16.0	
>= 2500	28	14,100	94	2.0	
	93	15,000	100		6.2

2. Hospital Group B: Hospitals with NICUs

Birthweight Strata	Deaths	Births	% of Total	Stratum Specific Rate per 1000	Crude Rate per 1000
< 1500	65	300	2	216.7	
1500 – 2499	14	1,200	8	11.7	
>= 2500	14	13,500	90	1.0	
	93	15,000	100		6.2

External Standard: All Live Births in the State

Birthweight Strata	Deaths	Births	% of Total	Stratum Specific Rate per 1000	Crude Rate per 1000
< 1500	1,375	5,000	1	275.0	
1500 – 2499	490	35,000	7	14.0	
>= 2500	460	460,000	92	1.0	
	2,325	500,000	100		4.65

The crude relative risk of neonatal death (not accounting for the birthweight distribution) when the two hospital groups are compared is 1 (6.2/6.2). Standardizing by birthweight will help determine if this relationship is a fair reflection of the neonatal mortality experience in the two hospital groups.

Standardization can be accomplished in two different ways:

Direct standardization applies the stratum specific rates of each population to the number of individuals in the corresponding stratum in the standard population. This method yields an adjusted relative risk. The method is called "direct" because it uses the actual morbidity or mortality rates of the populations being compared.

Indirect standardization, on the other hand, applies the stratum specific rates of the standard population to the number of individuals in the corresponding stratum in each of the populations being compared. This method is called "indirect" because nowhere does it use the actual morbidity or mortality rates of the populations being compared. Instead of an adjusted relative risk, indirect standardization yields standardized morbidity or mortality ratios (SMRs), one for each population being compared. Direct estimates are preferable to indirect ones, but the indirect method is used when the rates from the populations being compared are based on small numbers and therefore considered unreliable.

Direct Standardization

Using the numbers from the entire state and the rates for the two hospital groups shown in the hypothetical data above, a directly standardized relative risk is calculated as follows:

Adjusted Rate for the Community Hospitals:

$$= \frac{5,000 \times 353.3 + 35,000 \times 16.0 + 460,000 \times 2.0}{500,000}$$

$$= 6.5$$

Adjusted Rate for Tertiary Care Hospitals:

$$= \frac{5,000 \times 216.7 + 35,000 \times 11.7 + 460,000 \times 1.0}{500,000}$$

$$= 3.9$$

$$\text{Crude Relative Risk} = \frac{6.2}{6.2} = 1.0$$

$$\text{Standardized Relative Risk} = \frac{6.5}{3.9} = 1.7$$

In the process of calculating an adjusted relative risk, you can see that it is necessary to calculate what appear to be adjusted rates for each population. These recalculated rates, however, reflect what would be expected in the standard population if it had the morbidity or mortality experience of the populations being compared. In this example, the adjusted rates of 6.5 and 3.9, therefore, do not reflect the real mortality risk in the two hospital groups. They are byproducts of the standardization procedure and should not be used as stand-alone measures. In practice, these rates are sometimes reported despite the fact that they can lead to misleading and inappropriate conclusions.

The adjusted relative risk of 1.7 shows that the community hospitals have elevated neonatal mortality compared to the tertiary care centers even though the unadjusted relative risk was 1. Without adjustment, the better survival of neonates born in the tertiary care centers was masked due to the disparity in the birthweight distribution of the infants served by the two hospital groups; While the tertiary care centers have a higher incidence of low birthweight births than the community hospitals (10% v. 6 %), they have a lower neonatal mortality rate within each birthweight stratum (216.7 v. 353.0, 11.7 v.16.0, and 1.0 v. 2.0).

Indirect Standardization

Using the rates for the entire state and the numbers for the two hospital groups shown in the hypothetical data above, two standardized mortality ratios are calculated as follows:

For the Community Hospitals

$$SMR = \dfrac{\dfrac{93}{15,000} \times 1,000}{\dfrac{150 \times 275 + 750 \times 14.0 + 14,100 \times 1.0}{15,000}}$$

$$= \dfrac{6.2}{4.4}$$

$$= 1.4$$

For the Tertiary Care Centers

$$SMR = \dfrac{\dfrac{93}{15,000} \times 1,000}{\dfrac{300 \times 275 + 1,200 \times 14.0 + 13,500 \times 1.0}{15,000}}$$

$$= \dfrac{6.2}{7.5}$$

$$= 0.8$$

With indirect standardization, each SMR is itself an adjusted relative risk; the numerator is the observed crude rate in a population and the denominator is its expected rate given the neonatal mortality experience in the standard population. An SMR > 1 indicates higher rates than expected and an SMR < 1 indicates lower rates than expected. The two SMRs in this example lead to the same conclusion as did the adjusted relative risk—after accounting for birthweight the community hospitals have higher neonatal mortality than do the tertiary care centers.

It is not technically correct to create a ratio of two SMRs and interpret it as a relative risk; each SMR is itself a relative risk, and as such its value is compared to an expected value of 1. In practice, however, SMRs are sometimes compared in this fashion. In this example, the ratio of the two SMRs is 1.4/0.8 or 1.75, very similar to the value of 1.7 for the adjusted relative risk obtained from direct standardization.

Question:

The following table includes data from a hypothetical state survey that asked parents to report whether their children have a medical home. In addition, the table includes data from a county in the same state. The data are stratified by income level. Use indirect standardization to calculate an SMR that compares the county to the state with respect to the percent of children who have a medical home. Interpret the SMR.

Income Strata	# of Children with a Medical Home in the County	# of Children in the County	% of Children in the State Survey with a Medical Home
< $10,000	780	1,200	70.0
$10,000-$30,000	2,530	4,600	45.0
$30,000-$50,000	2,170	3,100	60.0
>$50,000	990	1,100	80.0
	6,470	10,000	

Answer:

$$SMR = \frac{\dfrac{6,470}{10,000} \times 100}{\dfrac{780 \times 70 + 2,530 \times 45 + 2,170 \times 60 + 990 \times 80}{10,000}}$$

$$= \frac{64.7}{56.5}$$

$$= 1.15$$

In this case, having a medical home is a positive, rather than an adverse outcome and therefore an SMR > 1 indicates that the children in this particular county are somewhat more likely to have a medical home than are children statewide.

Now that the process of direct and indirect standardization has been illustrated using a particular external standard, it is important to recognize that equivalent results would be obtained with some other external standard or even with an internal standard. For example, a national hospital data-set could have been used as an external standard, or one of the two hospital groups or the two hospital groups combined could have been used as an internal standard. While the choice of different standards will impact intermediate calculations, the adjusted relative risks or SMRs will all lead to the same interpretation. In fact, the adjusted relative risks from direct standardization will be the same regardless of the standard used.

The advantage of using a common external standard, either with direct or indirect standardization, is that many geographic areas and many time periods can be compared. For example, if the neonatal mortality rates of hospital groups in another region had been compared by standardizing for birthweight with the same statewide data as was used above, it would also be possible to compare the community hospitals across regions or the tertiary care hospitals across regions. If internal standards were used, the results for the two regions would not be immediately comparable.

Interestingly, stratified analysis as described in our earlier discussion of confounding and effect modification is equivalent to direct standardization with all of the observed data combined being the internal standard. For instance, following are the same hospital group data organized into a set of 2 × 2 tables for stratified analysis. There is one table for each birthweight stratum, the "exposure" is delivery in a community hospital v. delivery in a tertiary care center, and the outcome is neonatal death v. neonatal survivor.

Birthweight < 1,500 grams

		Neonatal Death Y	Neonatal Death N	
HOSP	A	53	97	150
HOSP	B	65	235	300
		118	332	450

Birthweight 1,500-2,499 grams

		Neonatal Death Y	Neonatal Death N	
HOSP	A	12	738	750
HOSP	B	14	1,186	1,200
		26	1,924	1,950

Birthweight >= 2,500 grams

Neonatal Death

		Y	N	
H A		28	14,072	14,100
O S				
P B		14	13,486	13,500
		42	27,558	27,600

$$RR_1 = \frac{353.3}{216.7} = 1.6$$

$$RR_2 = \frac{16.0}{11.7} = 1.4$$

$$RR_3 = \frac{2.0}{1.0} = 2.0$$

$$\text{Adj. } RR = 1.7$$

Notice that the estimate of the adjusted relative risk (1.7) is the same as that obtained from direct standardization using an external standard, underscoring the correspondence between the two methodologies. With the data organized in this fashion, however, the difference in the stratum specific estimates can also be seen. The process of rate standardization always assumes that a summary measure is appropriate to report, and while it is debatable as to whether effect modification exists in this example, the organization of the data for stratified analysis encourages closer examination of the stratum specific estimates. In this case, it is interesting to see that, the relative risk of neonatal death at the community hospitals compared to the tertiary care centers is actually highest in the normal birthweight category (2.0/1.0=2). While one would expect the community hospitals not to perform as well with high risk infants since they are not equipped to manage them, it is disturbing that their performance is also worse with low risk infants.

Too often, stratum specific information is ignored in favor of the adjusted summary measure. Sometimes this is deemed necessary if, for example, many indicators are being examined, and reporting all of the stratum specific rates may be providing an audience more information than can be easily absorbed. In this circumstance, reporting one summary measure for each indicator may do a better job of communicating a coherent picture of the health status of a population. On the other hand, when the public health focus is on more effective and efficient targeting of interventions and on prioritizing allocation of resources, stratum specific information may in fact be more useful than summary measures.

Moreover, it is important not to confuse the reporting of relative comparisons across populations with examining the true level of an outcome in each population. There is a temptation to try and do both simultaneously by reporting the adjusted rates obtained from the standardization process. A series of such rates implies comparisons across populations, but it also implies that each rate reflects the true level of the outcome in a population which, as was pointed out earlier, it does not. It is better to report an adjusted relative risk or SMR for comparison purposes and in addition report the actual observed stratum specific rates to give a sense of the occurrence of the outcome in each population. In the hospital group example, the adjusted relative risk of 1.7 could be reported along with the stratum specific neonatal mortality rates of 353.3, 16.0, and 2 per 1,000 live births for the community hospitals and then 216.7, 11.7, and 1.0 per 1,000 live births for the tertiary care centers.

Finally, remember that adjustment for confounding is not appropriate when the third factor is in the causal pathway. If the association of interest were smoking status and neonatal mortality instead of hospital group and neonatal mortality, it would be inappropriate to standardize for or stratify by birthweight since birthweight is in the causal path between smoking and neonatal mortality. This illustrates the importance of basing analytic choices on substantive and not mechanical grounds.

SYNTHETIC ESTIMATION

Simple synthetic estimation is part of the process of indirect standardization. Stratum specific rates from either population data, or from a large sample survey are applied to observed numbers in the population of interest. In other words, the denominator of an SMR is a synthetic estimate. This estimate is used when data for an indicator are not collected for the local area and therefore there is no observed value from the local area to use as a numerator for an SMR. A synthetic estimate may also be used when the direct data for the area are available, but known to be under or over-reported, or very unreliable due to small sample size.

Indirect estimates, including SMRs as well as synthetic estimates, are probably biased (in a statistical sense), but they are usually quite reliable since they are derived from very stable rates from large populations or surveys. Recalling that the accuracy of an estimate is dependent on both bias and reliability, using a somewhat biased synthetic estimate may be preferable to using very unstable direct data. And when no direct data are available, the choice is between using a synthetic estimate or none at all.

Suppose we did not have access to direct data for the two hospital groups used in the previous example of standardization, but a comparison of neonatal mortality in the two groups was still desired. If the same hypothetical standard—based on all live births in the State—were used to calculate separate synthetic estimates for the two hospital groups, the results would be:

$$\text{Synthetic Estimate}_A = 4.4$$

$$\text{Synthetic Estimate}_B = 7.5$$

These are the denominators of the SMRs calculated earlier or the expected rates in the two hospital groups (see page 96). By using the neonatal mortality experience in the State as a whole as the standard, the assumption is that it is a reasonable reflection of the neonatal mortality experience in each hospital group. Notice, however, that the synthetic estimate for Hospital Group A is lower than that for Hospital Group B, implying that the community hospitals have a better neonatal mortality rate than do the tertiary care centers. This contradicts the results of both direct and indirect standardization as well as the stratified analysis. This kind of result illustrates the danger of using synthetic estimates.

For synthetic estimation to be credible, then, it is critical to use a standard with strata that account for important characteristics of the population for which the estimate is being calculated. With no direct data as a basis of comparison, we must be confident that the stratum specific rates applied to the numbers in the population of interest are close to those that would be observed in that population. To calculate reasonable synthetic estimates for the tertiary care centers and community hospitals, for example, the standard would have to be stratified by hospital type as well as by birthweight—in effect, two distinct standards should be used. The data table for calculating the synthetic estimates would then be organized as follows, with 6 rather than 3 strata for the standard as well as for the hospital groups. Now, the synthetic estimates for the community hospitals can be calculated using only the rates from community hospitals statewide, and the synthetic estimate for the tertiary care centers can be calculated using only the rates from tertiary care centers statewide.

	# of Deaths in the Hospitals of Interest	# of Births in the Hospitals of Interest	Stratum Specific Rates from the Standard	Synthetic Estimates or Expected # of Deaths
Community Hospitals < 1500 1500 – 2499 >= 2500				
Tertiary Care Centers < 1500 1500 – 2499 >= 2500				

If an overall synthetic estimate for all hospitals in the region had been desired rather than separate estimates by hospital type, then using all live births in the state as the standard would have been appropriate. Combining the data for Hospital Group A and Hospital Group B into regional totals, we get:

Hospital Groups A and B Combined:

Birthweight	Deaths	Births	%	Stratum Specific Rates from the Standard per 1000	Crude Rate per 1000
< 1500	118	450	1.5	262.0	
1500 – 2499	26	1,950	6.5	13.0	
>= 2500	42	27,600	92.0	1.5	
	186	30,000	100.0		6.2

Remember that the crude rate in each of the hospital groups was 6.2 and therefore the combined crude rate is also 6.2. Multiplying the number of births in the birthweight strata in the above table by the neonatal mortality rates from the hypothetical standard, we get the following synthetic estimate:

$$\frac{450 \times 275 + 1,950 \times 14.0 + 27,600 \times 1.0}{30,000}$$

$$= 6.0$$

This synthetic estimate of 6.0 is a reasonable reflection of the actual crude rate in the two hospital groups combined, 6.2.

Following is another example of synthetic estimation. The standard is national survey data stratified on multiple variables to calculate an overall state synthetic estimate of the percent of women who drink alcohol during pregnancy. The strata chosen to calculate the estimate were African-American/Non African-American, married/not married, and age < 20, 20-34, and >= 35. Separate estimates for African-American and Non African-American women, or for women in specific age groups could also be calculated analogous to the separate estimates for the community and tertiary care hospitals.

Although direct data have been available on the birth certificate for alcohol use during pregnancy since 1989, it is likely that in the first few years of data collection, the error rate was high. These data are for 1989.

Strata	# of Drinkers Reported on the Birth Certificate	# of Live Births	Stratum Specific Percents of Alcohol Use During Pregnancy National Survey Data	Synthetic Estimates or Expected # of Drinkers
African-American				
< 20, Married	0	281	0.06	17
< 20, Not Married	99	10,396	0.07	728
20-34, Married	183	7,531	0.11	828
20-34, Not Married	972	18,003	0.16	2,880
> = 35, Married	33	1,002	0.11	110
> = 35, Not Married	77	896	0.13	116
Non African-American				
< 20, Married	38	4,264	0.14	597
< 20, Unmarried	134	8,873	0.09	799
20-34, Married	2,761	98,712	0.24	23,691
20-34, Not Married	701	16,083	0.24	3,860
> = 35, Married	584	12,401	0.24	2,976
> = 35, Not Married	67	942	0.25	236
Total	5,649	179,384		36,838

Direct Estimate from Birth Certificate = (5,649/179,384)*100 = 3.1

Synthetic Estimate = (36,838/179,384)*100 = 20.5

In this example, the synthetic estimate of 20.5 % is much higher than the 3.1 % reported in the birth certificate data. We hypothesize that there is underreporting in the birth certificate data, yet we may also not feel confident in the synthetic estimate. Other stratification schemes might be tried to assess any change in the resulting synthetic estimate. In addition, a small local survey may be undertaken in an attempt to get another estimate as a point of comparison.

Should we report either of these less than ideal estimates of alcohol use during pregnancy? Often, it is a matter of public health discretion whether to report estimates in which we do not have full confidence, either because they contain statistical or epidemiologic bias or because they are unreliable. The consequences for public health programs of reporting or not reporting such estimates must be considered. Ironically, there is often more comfort in reporting estimates that are known or suspected to be inaccurate if they are direct estimates, such as poorly reported indicators from vital records, than in reporting indirect (synthetic) estimates that in fact may be more accurate. MCH professionals need to bring their clinical and programmatic knowledge to bear when deciding which indicators are important and which estimates of those indicators to report.

Question:

Again using the hypothetical statewide data for the percent of children who have a medical home (See page 97 from Test Yourself), calculate a county synthetic estimate. Is it a reasonable estimate? Could its accuracy be increased?

Answer:

$$\text{Synthetic Estimate} = \frac{780 \times 70 + 2{,}530 \times 45 + 2{,}170 \times 60 + 990 \times 80}{10{,}000}$$

$$= 56.5$$

The synthetic estimate of 56.5 % is fairly close to the actual observed county percent of 64.7. A variable such as insurance status, (or other variables related to both county of residence and having a medical home) could be used to create additional strata in an effort to increase the accuracy of the synthetic estimate.

OVERVIEW OF MULTIVARIABLE REGRESSION METHODS

Regression analysis can be viewed as an alternative to as well as an extension of stratified analysis. Like stratified analysis, regression approaches allow examination of multiple factors (independent variables) simultaneously in relation to an outcome (dependent variable) and provide a means of controlling confounding and examining effect modification. Unlike stratified analysis, regression approaches can more efficiently handle many variables, and continuous as well as discrete variables can be analyzed.

The most common regression models used to analyze health data express the hypothesized association between risk or other factors and an outcome as a linear relationship. Ordinary Least Squares (OLS) regression is used when the outcome of interest is a continuous variable (or is close to continuous). Logistic regression is used most often when the outcome of interest is dichotomous.

A linear model in its simplest form is as follows:

$$E(\text{Outcome}) = \text{Intercept} + (\text{Slope} \times \text{risk factor})$$

where E stands for "Expected Value of"

When the outcome is a continuous, normally distributed variable, the values of the outcome variable are assumed to be linearly related to the values of a risk factor or other variable of interest. The model is written as follows:

$$E(Y) = a + (b \times \text{risk factor})$$

When the outcome is a dichotomous, binomially distributed variable, it is the *natural logarithm of the odds of the outcome* that is assumed to be linearly related to the values of a risk factor or other variable of interest. The model is written:

$$E\left(\ln\frac{p}{1-p}\right) = a + (b \times \text{risk factor})$$

When the outcome is a very small binomial variable, or Poisson distributed, it is the *natural logarithm of the rate of the outcome* that is assumed to be linearly related to the values of a risk factor or other variable of interest. The model is written:

$$E(\ln r) = a + (b \times \text{risk factor})$$

Regression models provide a more comprehensive approach to testing hypotheses about associations based on means and proportions. Recall that hypothesis tests are carried out in the following way:

$$\text{Test Statistic} = \frac{\text{Observed Association - Expected Association}}{\text{Standard Error of the Association}}$$

Previously, we expressed an observed association in terms of differences between means and proportions or as odds ratios and relative risks. These same measures of association are relevant in regression analysis, but now they are embodied in the slope of the regression line, or what is called the beta coefficient. The test statistic from regression analysis, then, is written:

$$\text{Test Statistic} = \frac{\text{Observed Slope(beta) - Expected Slope(beta)}}{\text{Standard Error of the Slope(beta)}}$$

The observed beta coefficient can theoretically range from negative infinity to positive infinity $(-\infty$ to $\infty)$, and its expected value under the assumption of no association (the null hypothesis) is 0. In OLS regression, with an outcome that is a continuous, normally distributed variable, the slope or beta coefficient is a measure of differences between means. In logistic regression, with an outcome that is a binomial proportion, the slope or beta coefficient is the odds ratio.

Regression models can be quite complicated, including many independent variables, both continuous and discrete. In this way, regression models attempt to capture the complex context in which health events occur. A more complicated linear regression model looks like:

$$E(\text{Outcome}) = \text{Intercept} + (\text{beta}_1 \times \text{factor}_1) + (\text{beta}_2 \times \text{factor}_2) + \Lambda + (\text{beta}_n \times \text{factor}_n)$$

Test statistics for each of the many beta coefficients may be of interest, or more typically, most of the variables are included as potential confounders or effect modifiers in order to insure appropriate adjustment of the beta coefficient for the variable of primary interest. Statistics that assess the strength of the entire model, or the association between all of the variables in the model jointly with the outcome may also be examined.

In addition to statistical testing, regression models can help us better describe the occurrence of a health outcome in a population in a multivariable context which, of course, better mirrors the multivariable world. Following are examples of different regression models with brief explanations of how the results might be interpreted. The examples illustrate inclusion of different types of variables as well as how to substitute values into the regression equation to obtain useful, reportable estimates. In the examples of OLS regression, estimates of means and then mean differences are shown; in the examples of logistic regression, estimates of odds and then odds ratios are shown. The numbers in these examples are hypothetical, based only loosely on what might be found in the MCH literature.

First, here are some examples using ordinary least squares regression:

Example 1: Birthweight is the outcome variable measured continuously in grams, adequacy of prenatal care (PNC) is the independent variable measured dichotomously with women who received no or inadequate PNC coded 1 and those who received adequate PNC coded 0.

$$E(\text{birthweight in grams}) = 3,150 + (-250 \times \text{PNC})$$

On average, the birthweight of infants born to women who received no or inadequate prenatal care is estimated to be:

$$3,150 - 250(1) = 2,900 \text{ grams}$$

On average, the birthweight of infants born to women who received adequate prenatal care is estimated to be:

$$3,150 - 250(0) = 3,150 \text{ grams}$$

In this case, the beta coefficient is a measure of the difference in mean birthweight among women with varying patterns of prenatal care utilization. Infant birthweight among women who received no or inadequate prenatal care is 250 grams less, on average, than infant birthweight among women who received adequate prenatal care. The standard error of the beta coefficient can be used to calculate a confidence interval around this value of 250 grams, and depending on whether this confidence interval includes 0, the associated p value will indicate whether this mean difference is statistically significant.

Example 2: Birthweight is the outcome variable measured continuously in grams, adequacy of prenatal care is the independent variable measured continuously in number of visits.

$$E(\text{birthweight in grams}) = 3{,}150 + (12 \times \# \text{ of prenatal care visits})$$

On average, the birthweight of infants born to women who received 10 prenatal care visits is estimated to be:

$$3{,}150 + 12(10) = 3{,}270 \text{ grams}$$

On average, the birthweight of infants born to women who received 5 prenatal care visits is estimated to be:

$$3{,}150 + 12(5) = 3{,}210 \text{ grams}$$

On average, the birthweight of infants born to women who received no prenatal care is estimated to be:

$$3{,}150 + 12(0) = 3{,}150 \text{ grams}$$

As before, the beta coefficient is a measure of the difference in mean birthweight, but now the difference can be assessed for each single additional prenatal care visit. For each visit, infant birthweight increases, on average, by an estimated 12 grams. Also as before, a standard error of the beta coefficient can be used to calculate a confidence interval around this value of 12 grams, and depending on whether this confidence interval includes 0, the associated p value will indicate whether this mean difference is statistically significant.

When continuous variables such as number of prenatal care visits are included in a linear regression model, the assumption is that the association between the independent and dependent variable is the same across all of the values of the independent variable. In the above example, it is assumed that each additional prenatal care visit adds equivalent benefit; the change in infant birthweight if a woman receives 10 versus 9 prenatal care visits is the same as the change if a woman receives 2 versus 1 prenatal care visit. For many variables used in maternal and child health, this may not be a valid assumption.

Consider maternal AGE as a variable of interest in studying perinatal outcomes. Women who deliver at a very young age and women who deliver at ages over 35 are usually considered at higher risk of adverse outcomes than other women. In order to capture this non-linear relationship in a regression model, "dummy" variables are coded. These are a set of dichotomous variables, coded "1" and "0", that jointly represent the effect of age.

Suppose 3 categories of maternal AGE are to be examined:

< 18
18-34
35 +

In order to examine these categories in a regression model, the following 2 "dummy" variables would be created:

AGE	LESS18	PLUS35
< 18	1	0
18-34	0	0
35+	0	1

Notice that the number of "dummy" variables coded is equal to one less than the number of categories of interest. Here, the 3 categories of AGE are fully defined with 2 "dummy" variables. The variable value which is coded "0" on each "dummy" is called the reference group; here, it is the women who are 18-34. This is the comparison group for all odds ratios pertaining to age.

A similar categorization scheme may be called for when considering prenatal care visits. Women with very few and very many prenatal care visits may be at higher risk for delivering a low birthweight infant. The following dummy variables might be used in a regression model to address this situation:

# OF PRENATAL CARE VISITS	LESS5	PLUS12
< 5	1	0
5-12	0	0
> 12	0	1

Let's examine what might occur in a regression model employing these dummy variables for prenatal care visits.

Example 3: Birthweight is the outcome variable measured continuously in grams, prenatal care is the independent variable measured with two dummy variables coded as in the above table.

$$E(\text{birthweight in grams}) = 3{,}150 + (-240 \times \text{LESS5}) + (-70 \times \text{PLUS12})$$

On average, the birthweight of infants born to women who received fewer than 5 prenatal care visits is estimated to be:
$$3{,}150 - 240(1) - 70(0) = 2{,}910 \text{ grams}$$

On average, the birthweight of infants born to women who received from 5-12 prenatal care visits is estimated to be:
$$3{,}150 - 240(0) - 70(0) = 3{,}150 \text{ grams}$$

On average, the birthweight of infants born to women who received more than 12 prenatal care visits is estimated to be:
$$3{,}150 - 240(0) - 70(1) = 3{,}080 \text{ grams}$$

The first beta coefficient (LESS5) is a measure of the difference in mean birthweight between women with fewer than 5 prenatal care visits compared to women with 5-12 visits; the second beta coefficient (PLUS12) is a measure of the difference in mean birthweight between women with more than 12 prenatal care visits compared to women with 5-12 visits. Infant birthweight among women who received fewer than 5 visits is 240 grams less, on average, than infant birthweight among women who received 5-12 visits. Infant birthweight among women who received more than 12 visits is 70 grams less, on average, than infant birthweight among women who received 5-12 visits. The standard errors of the beta coefficients can be used to calculate confidence intervals around the values of 240 and 70. Depending on whether these confidence intervals include 0, the associated p values will indicate whether these mean differences are statistically significant.

Comment and Example

Use of "dummy" variables is important because it permits inclusion of many categorical variables in a regression model without assuming a linear relationship. Suppose we want to assess the differences in mean number of well child visits received by two-year-olds in a three county region. The counties could be coded as follows:

County	VARXZ	VARYZ
X	1	0
Y	0	1
Z	0	0

The first dummy variable is named "VARXZ" to indicate that County X is coded 1 and County Z is the reference group; likewise, the second dummy variable is named "VARYZ" to indicate that County Y is coded 1 and again County Z is the reference group. A regression model of interest might be:

Dependent Variable: # well child visits

Independent Variables:

1. VARXZ
2. VARYZ
3. # pediatricians per child pop. in the county
4. Insurance Status (yes/no)

The results of this model would help answer questions about whether there are any differences in the amount of well child care being received by children in the three counties after accounting for differences in the supply of pediatricians and the insurance status of the children.

Next, here are a few examples using a logistic regression model:

Example 4: Birthweight is the outcome variable measured dichotomously with low birthweight (LBW) coded 1 and normal birthweight coded 0, prenatal care is the independent variable measured dichotomously with women who received no or inadequate PNC coded 1 and those who received adequate PNC coded 0.

$$E(\ln \text{ odds of LBW}) = -2.80 + (0.47 \times PNC)$$

On average, the odds of delivering a low birthweight infant among women whom received no or inadequate prenatal care is estimated to be:

$$e^{-2.80 + 0.47(1)} = 0.097$$

On average, the odds of delivering a low birthweight infant among women who received adequate prenatal care is estimated to be:

$$e^{-2.80 + 0.47(0)} = 0.061$$

The odds ratio for the association between prenatal care and low birthweight is estimated to be:

$$\frac{e^{-2.80+0.47(1)}}{e^{-2.80+0.47(0)}} = e^{0.47(1-0)} = 1.6$$

Here, you can see that when variables are coded "1" and "0", the beta coefficient itself is a measure of the natural logarithm of the odds ratio. On average, women who received no or inadequate prenatal care are 1.6 times more likely to deliver a low birthweight infant than are women who received adequate prenatal care. The standard error of the beta coefficient can be used to calculate a confidence interval around the value of 0.47 which when exponentiated yields a confidence interval around the value of 1.6. Depending on whether this confidence interval includes 1, the associated p value will indicate whether this odds ratio is statistically significant.

Example 5: Birthweight is the outcome variable measured dichotomously with low birthweight coded 1 and normal birthweight coded 0, prenatal care is the independent variable measured with two dummy variables coded as in the above table.

$$E(\ln \text{ odds of LBW}) = -2.80 + (0.53 \times \text{LESS5}) + (0.28 \times \text{PLUS12})$$

On average, the odds of delivering a lbw infant among women who received fewer than 5 prenatal care visits is estimated to be:

$$e^{-2.80 + 0.53(1) + 0.28(0)} = 0.10$$

On average, the odds of delivering a lbw infant among women who received 5-12 prenatal care visits is estimated to be:

$$e^{-2.80 + 0.53(0) + 0.28(0)} = 0.06$$

On average, the odds of delivering a lbw infant among women who received more than 12 prenatal care visits is estimated to be:

$$e^{-2.80 + 0.53(0) + 0.28(1)} = 0.08$$

The odds ratio for the association between receiving fewer than 5 visits versus 5-12 visits and low birthweight is estimated to be:

$$\frac{e^{-2.80+0.53(1)+0.28(0)}}{e^{-2.80+0.53(0)+0.28(0)}} = e^{0.53(1-0)} = 1.7$$

The odds ratio for the association between receiving more than 12 visits versus 5-12 visits and low birthweight is estimated to be:

$$\frac{e^{-2.80+0.53(0)+0.28(1)}}{e^{-2.80+0.53(0)+0.28(0)}} = e^{0.28(1-0)} = 1.3$$

The first beta coefficient (LESS5) is a measure of the natural logarithm of the odds ratio for women with fewer than 5 prenatal care visits compared to women with 5-12 visits; the second beta coefficient (PLUS12) is a measure of the natural logarithm of the odds ratio for women with more than 12 prenatal care visits compared to women with 5-12 visits. On average, women who received fewer than 5 visits are 1.7 times more likely to deliver a low birthweight infant than are women who received 5-12 visits; on average, women who received more than 12 visits are 1.3 times more likely to deliver a low birthweight infant than are women who received 5-12 visits. The standard errors of the beta coefficients can be used to calculate confidence intervals around the values of 0.53 and 0.28 which when exponentiated yield confidence intervals around the values of 1.7 and 1.3. Depending on whether these confidence intervals include 1, the associated p values will indicate whether these odds ratios are statistically significant.

If a continuous variable is to be used in a logistic regression model, an increase or decrease in the odds ratio for each single unit change in such a variable is usually not meaningful. For example, suppose we felt comfortable using number of prenatal care visits in its continuous form. The resulting beta coefficient from a logistic regression model might be 0.049, yielding an odds ratio for each additional prenatal visit of e^b or $e^{0.049} = 1.05$. This is not a readily interpretable result. Typically with a continuous variable, odds ratios are calculated for what is considered to be clinically or programmatically meaningful. An odds ratio might be calculated for a 5 visit difference, for instance, $e^{b(5)}$ or $e^{0.049\,(5)} = 1.28$.

Example 6: Birthweight is the outcome variable measured dichotomously with low birthweight coded 1 and normal birthweight coded 0, adequacy of prenatal care is the first independent variable measured dichotomously with women who received no or inadequate prenatal care coded 1 and women who received adequate care coded 0, and smoking status during pregnancy (SMOKE) is a second independent variable measured dichotomously with smokers coded 1 and nonsmokers coded 0.

$$E(\ln \text{ odds of LBW}) = -2.80 + (0.35 \times \text{PNC}) + (0.60 \times \text{SMOKE}) + (0.04 \times \text{PNC} \times \text{SMOKE})$$

In addition to the two independent variables for adequacy of prenatal care and smoking status, the model also includes a third variable that is the multiplication of these other two. This variable is called an interaction term and permits assessment of whether there is effect modification. Below are the possible combinations of values on the three variables in the model:

Coding of Variables

	PNC	SMOKE	PNC×SMOKE
Women with no/inadequate pnc who smoke	1	1	1
Women with adequate pnc who smoke	0	1	0
Women with no/inadequate pnc who do not smoke	1	0	0
Women with adequate pnc who do not smoke	0	0	0

On average, the odds of delivering a lbw infant among women who received no or inadequate prenatal care and smoked during pregnancy is estimated to be:

$$e^{-2.80 + 0.35(1) + 0.60(1) + 0.04(1)} = 0.16$$

On average, the odds of delivering a lbw infant among women who received adequate prenatal care and smoked during pregnancy is estimated to be:

$$e^{-2.80 + 0.35(0) + 0.60(1) + 0.04(0)} = 0.11$$

On average, the odds of delivering a lbw infant among women who received no or inadequate prenatal care and did not smoke during pregnancy is estimated to be:

$$e^{-2.80 + 0.35(1) + 0.60(0) + 0.04(0)} = 0.086$$

On average, the odds of delivering a lbw infant among women who received adequate prenatal care and did not smoke during pregnancy is estimated to be:

$$e^{-2.80 + 0.35(0) + 0.60(0) + 0.04(0)} = 0.06$$

On average, the odds ratio for the association between no or inadequate prenatal care and lbw among women who smoked during pregnancy is estimated to be:

$$\frac{e^{-2.80 + 0.35(1) + 0.60(1) + 0.04(1)}}{e^{-2.80 + 0.35(0) + 0.60(1) + 0.04(0)}} = e^{0.35(1-0) + 0.04(1-0)} = 1.48$$

On average, the odds ratio for the association between no or inadequate prenatal care and lbw among women who did not smoke during pregnancy is estimated to be:

$$\frac{e^{-2.80 + 0.35(1) + 0.60(0) + 0.04(0)}}{e^{-2.80 + 0.35(0) + 0.60(0) + 0.04(0)}} = e^{0.35(1-0)} = 1.42$$

When an interaction term (the variable assessing effect modification) is in a model, the meaning of each beta coefficient is not so straightforward. The first odds ratio above, for example, is determined by both the value of the beta coefficient for the prenatal care variable as well as the beta coefficient for the prenatal care by smoking variable. Likewise, the standard error and the test of statistical significance for this association is based on information from both the prenatal care variable and the prenatal care by smoking variable. These more complicated calculations are required because, by definition, the presence of effect modification requires the use of stratum specific estimates rather than a simpler summary measure.

To make the regression results easier to interpret when effect modification is present, often the analysis is stratified. In this example, two separate regression models could be run, one including only women who smoked during pregnancy, the other including only women who did not smoke during pregnancy. Now, prenatal care would be the only independent variable in each model, and its beta coefficient could be interpreted in the straightforward way it was in the earlier examples.

If there is no effect modification, as in this example with the equivalent stratum specific odds ratios of 1.48 and 1.42, stratified analysis is unnecessary and the interaction term can be removed from the model. If one regression model is used including both prenatal care and smoking, then the beta coefficient for prenatal care (after exponentiation) is the odds ratio for the association between adequacy of prenatal care and low birthweight adjusted for the effect of smoking. The model might look like:

$$E(\ln \text{ odds of LBW}) = -2.80 + (0.37 \times \text{PNC}) + (0.62 \times \text{SMOKE})$$

The association of adequacy of prenatal care and low birthweight adjusted for the effect of smoking is $e^{0.37} = 1.44$. For these data, then, smoking is a confounder since the crude odds ratio was 1.6 as seen earlier (page 109).

Comment

Stratified analysis is analogous to the logistic regression model. For this example, the 2 × 2 tables would be:

Smokers

Low Birthweight

		Y	N
No or Inadequate PNC	Y		
	N		

Non-Smokers

Low Birthweight

		Y	N
No or Inadequate PNC	Y		
	N		

Question:

Following are hypothetical results of a logistic regression model for examining adolescent suicide in relation to age and gender. Suicide is a dichotomous variable, 1=yes, 0=no. Age is a dichotomous variable, 1=20-21 years old, 0=15-19 years old. Gender is a dichotomous variable, 1=male, 0=female. What is the odds ratio for the association between gender and suicide after adjusting for the effect of age? Interpret this result.

$$E(\ln \text{ odds of committing suicide}) = -9.7 + 0.1 \times \text{age} + 1.3 \times \text{gender}$$

Answer:

OR=$e^{1.3}$=3.7. On average male adolescents are 3.7 times more likely to commit suicide than female adolescents.

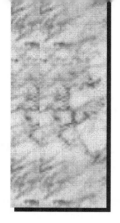

Epidemiology and Biostatistics
Exercises and Solutions

Rates and Percent Distributions

Exercise A

The following are data for two counties:

County	Total Pop	Total Births	Total Females Ages 15-44	Total Females Ages 10-17	Births Ages 10-17
X	317,471	6,289	80,168	20,422	278
Y	182,827	2,808	56,869	16,869	213

Recall the formulas for the crude birth and fertility rates:

Crude Birth Rate

$$\frac{\text{Total Births}}{\text{Total Population}} \times 1,000$$

Crude Fertility Rate

$$\frac{\text{Total Births}}{\text{Females Ages 15 - 44}} \times 1,000$$

For each of the counties, calculate the following:

1. the crude birth rate

2. the crude fertility rate

3. the fertility rate for adolescents aged 10-17

4. the percent of total births to adolescents aged 10-17

Do either County X or County Y have an excess of adolescent births? Which county is in more need of programs targeted at the adolescent population?

Prevalence vs. Incidence

Exercise B

In June, 1995, at the end of their senior year, the following observations were made concerning smoking in a population of 110 graduating seniors. The enrollment for this cohort from 9th to 12th grade was as follows:

9th	Sept. 1991	160
10th	Sept. 1992	140
11th	Sept. 1993	120
12th	Sept. 1994	110

The seniors were asked the following question. "At any time while you were in high school (Sept. '91 - June '95), did you smoke at least one pack of cigarettes a week? If yes, when did you start and for how long did you smoke?" Of the 110 graduating seniors surveyed, 20 reported having smoked at some time during high school. The following table shows the data for these 20 students:

Student	Started Smoking	Quit Smoking
1	Oct. 1, '89	Still smoking
2	Nov. 1, '92	July 31, '94
3	Dec. 1, '94	Still smoking
4	Oct. 1, '91	Aug. 31, '92
(Student 4 cont.)	Sept. 1, '93	Aug. 31, '94
5	Sept. 1, '94	Sept. 30, '94
6	Feb. 1, '92	Still smoking
7	Jan. 1, '90	Dec. 31, '93
8	Sept. 1, '92	Nov. 30, '94
9	Jan. 1, '94	Still smoking
10	Sept. 1, '91	Aug. 31, '94
11	Sept. 1, '92	Aug. 31, '94
12	Feb. 1, '90	Still smoking
13	July 1, '92	Sept. 30, '92
14	Aug. 1, '93	Aug 31, '93
15	Sept. 1, '94	Still smoking
16	Jan. 1, '94	Still smoking
17	Sept. 1, '92	Sept. 30, '92
18	Sept. 1, '91	Still smoking
19	Sept. 1, '92	Aug. 31, '94
20	Sept. 1, '94	Still smoking

Graphically, the smoking status of these 20 students can be depicted as follows:

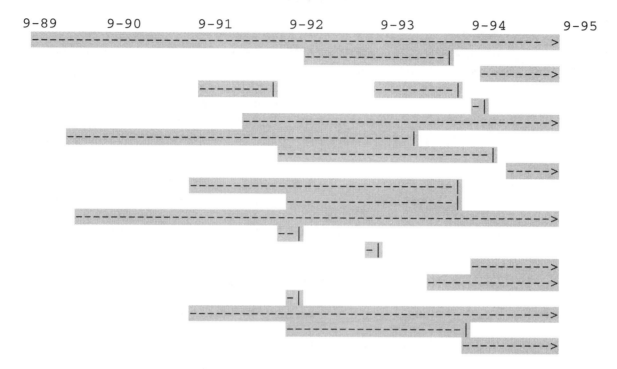

Using the data above, answer the following questions:

1. From Sept. 1993 - Aug. 31, 1994 what was the incidence rate of smoking?

2. What was the prevalence of smoking at the time of the survey in June, 1995?

3. The survey was given to the 110 graduating seniors. How valid are the results of the survey as estimates of smoking incidence and prevalence for the high school age adolescents in this community?

Incidence and Prevalence

Exercise C

The County Y Head Start Program enrolled 500 children in the Fall of 1995. All of these children were screened for vision problems at the beginning of the year and 50 were found to have vision problems.

When the same 500 children are screened again in the Fall of 1996, 65 are found to have vision problems.

1. What was the prevalence of vision problems in County Y's Head Start program in 1995?

2. What was the prevalence of vision problems in County Y's Head Start program in 1996?

3. What is the risk of developing vision problems between the Fall of 1995 and the Fall of 1996 in this group of Head Start children?

Incidence and Prevalence

Exercise D

The Hospital X Emergency Room in Community A recorded 120 asthma cases during 1995 out of a total of 1450 individual children seen. The state Children with Special Health Care Needs (CSHCN) program was interested in determining if these numbers meant an increased risk of a child developing asthma in Community A or a possible decrease in the effectiveness of the medication taken by asthmatic children in Community A. In 1996 they asked the hospital to track the number of first time asthma diagnoses admitted to the ER versus those asthma cases who visited the ER but had been previously diagnosed as having asthma.

In 1996 out of 1370 children seen in the ER, there were 130 asthma cases: 42 were new cases, 88 had been previously diagnosed prior to the ER visit.

1. What was the risk of having asthma in 1995 for children in Community A seeking ER care at Hospital X?

2. What was the prevalence of childhood asthma in 1995 in the ER at Hospital X in Community A?

3. What was the prevalence of childhood asthma in 1996 in the ER at Hospital X in Community A?

4. Can the state CSHCN program answer its question?

5. Does knowing the incidence of childhood asthma diagnoses in the ER at Hospital X in Community A in 1996 help? What is the incidence?

6. What else is needed to answer the CSHCN program's question?

Confidence Intervals and Hypothesis Testing

Exercise E

Here are some data for 1990 and 1995:

Births	Deaths	Year	Infant Mortality Rate per 1000
8,717	141	1990	16.2
5,673	74	1995	13.0

1. Calculate a 95% confidence interval around each of the two infant mortality rates.

2. Arrange the above data as a complete 2 × 2 data table to conform with the setup as shown on page 50. What is the exposure? What is the outcome?

3. Conduct a statistical test for the difference between two proportions. Are the two infant mortality rates significantly different at $p < 0.05$?

Confidence Intervals and Hypothesis Testing

Exercise F

The immunization rates at age 2 in two health service regions in the state, and the corresponding Year 2000 Objective are as follows:

	Survey Based Immunization Rate (%)	Year 2000 Objective (%)
Region 1	87.3	90
Region 2	79.4	

In region 1, the rate is based on 345 surveys; in Region 2, the rate is based on 726 surveys.

1. Calculate and report a 95% confidence limit around each of the estimates of the immunization rate.

2. Test and report whether the immunization rates are significantly different from each other.

3. Test and report whether each of the immunization rates is significantly different from the Year 2000 Objective of 90% of 2-year-old children having been appropriately immunized.

Preventive Fraction

Exercise G

The table below has data for a hypothetical population of 10,000 children, only 50 % of whom are in car seats. The overall motor vehicle injury rate is 70 per 10,000 children.

1. What is the incidence of motor vehicle injury among children who are in care seats? What is the incidence of motor vehicle injury among children who are not in car seats?

2. What is the preventive fraction or the program effectiveness? Using the preventive fraction, how many motor vehicle injuries in this population could be prevented if all children were in car seats?

3. Suppose the state health agency wants to know what the motor vehicle injury rate would be if the prevalence of car seat use could be raised from 50 % to 75 %. Rearrange the 2 × 2 table, and calculate the estimated overall injury rate.

		Motor Vehicle Injury		
		Yes	No	
Car Seat Use	Yes	20	4,980	5,000
	No	50	4,950	5,000
		70	9,930	10,000

Ecologic Analysis

Exercise H

In public health, aggregate data may be useful for looking at the relationship between health services and health status. Following is a 2 × 2 table that examines the county level association between supply of family practitioners and pediatricians and the Year 2000 Objective for two year old immunization status:

		% Complete Immunizations at Age 2		
		< 90%	>= 90%	
Primary Care Physicians	0 or < 5	5	10	15
per 10,000 Children	>= 5	5	30	35
		10	40	50

The data are for 50 hypothetical counties, 15 of which have either no primary care physicians with an office in the county or fewer than 5 per 10,000 children, and 10 of which are not meeting the Year 2000 Objective of 90% complete immunization at age two. Some of the relevant statistics for these data are:

$$p_1 = \frac{5}{15} = 0.33$$

$$p_2 = \frac{5}{35} = 0.14$$

$$\text{Outcome Prevalence: } p_0 = \frac{10}{50} = 0.20$$

$$\text{"Exposure" Prevalence: } \frac{15}{50} = 0.30$$

Calculate the relative prevalence (RP) and the population attributable risk % (PAR%) and comment on the interpretation of these measures.

Multivariable Analysis

Exercise I

The following table displays information about pediatric emergency room visits and hospitalizations by source of payment in three counties:

County		Children <18 Years Old		
		Population	**Hospital Admissions**	**ER Admissions**
P	Medicaid	9,303	1,385	108
	Non Medicaid	17,787	1,799	92
Q	Medicaid	16,563	2,790	207
	Non Medicaid	30,942	1,758	82
R	Medicaid	32,187	3,302	675
	Non Medicaid	42,622	1,859	366
Total				
	Medicaid	58,053	7,477	990
	Non Medicaid	91,351	5,416	540

You are interested in exploring whether there is an association between payment source and hospital or ER admission.

1. Arrange the data into the appropriate 2 × 2 tables to assess the crude (unadjusted) association between payment source and emergency room or hospital admissions for all three counties combined. What is the crude association between payment source and emergency room admissions? What is the crude association between payment source and hospital admissions? How similar are they?

2. Now you are interested in examining the association between payment source and ER and hospital admissions controlling for county of residence. Output from conducting this analysis in Epi-Info is provided. Payment source is the exposure variable (Medicaid, Non-Medicaid), Disease is either ER admissions or hospital admissions.

   a. What is the adjusted (weighted) relative risk between payment source and emergency room admissions controlling for county of residence?

   b. What is the adjusted (weighted) relative risk between payment source and hospital admissions controlling for county of residence?

   c. Is county of residence an effect modifier of the association between payment source and ER or hospital admissions?

   d. Is county of residence a confounder of the association between payment source and emergency room or hospital admissions?

ASSOCIATION BETWEEN PAYMENT SOURCE AND ER ADMISSIONS
CONTROLLING FOR COUNTY OF RESIDENCE

COUNTY P

```
        + Disease -                        Analysis of Single Table
    +--------+--------+                 Odds ratio = 2.26 (1.69 <OR< 3.01)
  +|   108  |  9195  |  9303          Cornfield 95% confidence limits for OR
    +--------+--------+                Relative risk = 2.24 (1.70 <RR< 2.96)
  -|    92  | 17695  | 17787         Taylor Series 95% confidence limits for RR
    +--------+--------+                Ignore relative risk if case control study.
  E    200    26890    27090
  x                                              Chi-Squares    P-values
  p                                             -----------    --------
  o                               Uncorrected    :    34.54     0.0000000  ---
  s                               Mantel-Haenszel:    34.53     0.0000000  ---
  u                               Yates corrected:    33.66     0.0000000  ---
  r
  e
```

COUNTY Q

```
     + Disease -
 +--------+--------+
+|   207  | 16356  | 16563
 +--------+--------+
-|    82  | 30860  | 30942
 +--------+--------+
E    289    47216    47505
x
p
o
s
u
r
e
```

Odds ratio = 4.76 (3.66 <OR< 6.21)
Cornfield 95% confidence limits for OR
Relative risk = 4.72 (3.65 <RR< 6.09)
Taylor Series 95% confidence limits for RR
Ignore relative risk if case control study.

	Chi-Squares	P-values
	-----------	--------
Uncorrected :	173.02	0.0000000 ---
Mantel-Haenszel:	173.02	0.0000000 ---
Yates corrected:	171.40	0.0000000 ---

COUNTY R

```
     + Disease -
 +--------+--------+
+|   675  | 31512  | 32187
 +--------+--------+
-|   366  | 42256  | 42622
 +--------+--------+
E   1041    73768    74809
x
p
o
s
u
r
e
```

Odds ratio = 2.47 (2.17 <OR< 2.82)
Cornfield 95% confidence limits for OR
Relative risk = 2.44 (2.15 <RR< 2.77)
Taylor Series 95% confidence limits for RR
Ignore relative risk if case control study.

	Chi-Squares	P-values
	-----------	--------
Uncorrected :	204.96	0.0000000 ---
Mantel-Haenszel:	204.96	0.0000000 ---
Yates corrected:	204.06	0.0000000 ---

ASSOCIATION BETWEEN PAYMENT SOURCE AND ER ADMISSIONS
CONTROLLING FOR COUNTY OF RESIDENCE

***** Stratified Analysis *****
Summary of 3 Tables

Crude odds ratio for all strata = 2.92
Mantel-Haenszel Weighted Odds Ratio = 2.74
Cornfield 95% Confidence Limits
2.48 < 2.74 < 3.07
Mantel-Haenszel Summary Chi Square = 382.99
P value = 0.00000000

Crude RR for all strata = 2.88
Mantel-Haenszel Weighted Relative Risk
of Disease, given Exposure = 2.71
Greenland/Robins Confidence Limits =
2.44 < MHRR < 3.01

ASSOCIATION BETWEEN PAYMENT SOURCE AND HOSPITAL ADMISSIONS
CONTROLLING FOR COUNTY OF RESIDENCE

COUNTY P

```
        + Disease -
     +--------+--------+
    +| 1385   | 7918   |  9303
     +--------+--------+
    -| 1799   | 15988  |  17787
     +--------+--------+
E    3184     23906      27090
x
p
o
s
u
r
e
```

Analysis of Single Table
Odds ratio = 1.55 (1.44 <OR< 1.68)
Cornfield 95% confidence limits for OR
Relative risk = 1.47 (1.38 <RR< 1.57)
Taylor Series 95% confidence limits for RR
Ignore relative risk if case control study.

	Chi-Squares	P-values
Uncorrected :	134.19	0.0000000 ---
Mantel-Haenszel:	134.19	0.0000000 ---
Yates corrected:	133.74	0.0000000 ---

COUNTY Q

```
        + Disease -
     +--------+--------+
    +| 2790   | 13733  |  16523
     +--------+--------+
    -| 1758   | 29184  |  30942
     +--------+--------+
E    4548     42917      47465
x
p
o
s
u
r
e
```

Odds ratio = 3.37 (3.17 <OR< 3.59)
Cornfield 95% confidence limits for OR
Relative risk = 2.97 (2.81 <RR< 3.15)
Taylor Series 95% confidence limits for RR
Ignore relative risk if case control study.

	Chi-Squares	P-values
Uncorrected :	1560.64	0.0000000 ---
Mantel-Haenszel:	1560.61	0.0000000 ---
Yates corrected:	1559.35	0.0000000 ---

COUNTY R

```
        + Disease -
     +--------+--------+
    +| 3302   | 28885  |  32187
     +--------+--------+
    -| 1859   | 40763  |  42622
     +--------+--------+
E    5161     69648      74809
x
p
o
s
u
r
e
```

Odds ratio = 2.51 (2.36 <OR< 2.66)
Cornfield 95% confidence limits for OR
Relative risk = 2.35 (2.23 <RR< 2.48)
Taylor Series 95% confidence limits for RR
Ignore relative risk if case control study.

	Chi-Squares	P-values
Uncorrected :	992.93	0.0000000 ---
Mantel-Haenszel:	992.91	0.0000000 ---
Yates corrected:	992.01	0.0000000 ---

ASSOCIATION BETWEEN PAYMENT SOURCE AND HOSPITAL ADMISSIONS
CONTROLLING FOR COUNTY OF RESIDENCE

```
***** Stratified Analysis *****
         Summary of 3 Tables

Crude odds ratio for all strata =  2.35
Mantel-Haenszel Weighted Odds Ratio =  2.47
      Cornfield 95% Confidence Limits
         2.38 <  2.47 <  2.57
Mantel-Haenszel Summary Chi Square = 2423.97
         P value = 0.00000000


Crude RR for all strata =  2.17
Mantel-Haenszel Weighted Relative Risk
   of Disease, given Exposure =  2.27
   Greenland/Robins Confidence Limits =
         2.20 < MHRR <  2.35
```

3. Suggest two other variables that might be important in more precisely characterizing the relationship between payment source and ER and hospital admissions. Describe possible regression models that include county of residence, payment source and the new variables you identify.

   What type of regression procedures would you use (linear-ordinary least squares or linear logistic)?

   Would the variables in the models be continuous or categorical? Describe the coding for each variable.

Synthetic Estimation

Exercise J

The State health department wants to assist counties in examining data on weight, diet, and exercise in high school age youth. It provides counties with tables from the statewide Youth Risk Behavior Survey so that local synthetic estimates pertaining to these issues can be calculated.

The state provides estimates by age for black and white youth only as there were fewer than 100 youth in other racial/ethnic designations. Following are the state survey results for Question 64 on the survey which asks, "How do you describe your weight?" The results are percentages of respondents who described themselves as slightly or very overweight.

Weighted Percentages from the State Youth Risk Behavior Survey
Question 64: How do you describe your weight?

Age	Total	Black	White
<= 15	29.0	26.2	29.3
16 - 17	27.0	25.7	27.4
Total	**28.4**	**25.9**	**28.5**

The following table shows the numbers of high school age youth in County X stratified by age and racial designation. County X calculates a synthetic estimate considering the same strata as provided in the state results.

High School Age Youth in County X

Age	Total	Black	White
<= 15	936	172	764
16 - 17	811	130	681
Total	**1,747**	**302**	**1,445**

1. Calculate a synthetic estimate for County X of the number and percent of high school age youth who describe themselves as being slightly or very overweight. Report the stratum specific expected numbers of youth as well as the overall number and percent.

2. How similar or different are the synthetic county estimates from the State estimates?

3. What factors might determine whether County X considers the synthetic estimate appropriate for use in public health decision making?

4. How might the county estimates be improved? What might the State do to further assist counties in obtaining appropriate estimates?

Interpreting Regression Results

Exercise K

Results of a logistic regression analysis exploring the relationship between maternal characteristics and risk of postneonatal death among low risk infants are shown below. Low risk was defined as an infant whose birthweight was greater or equal to 2500 grams and whose gestational age was greater than or equal to 37 weeks.

The crude postneonatal mortality rate among low risk black infants was 4.5 per 1000; the crude postneonatal mortality rate among low risk white infants was 2 per 1000. The data are from 2 years of vital records from the ten states in federal regions V and VII

Table I: Select Maternal Characteristics and the Odds of Postneonatal Death Among Low Risk Infants

Variables	Black (N = 124,988)		White (N = 889,311)	
Age/Education	**Odds Ratio**	**95% Confidence Interval**	**Odds Ratio**	**95% Confidence Interval**
10 - 19 yrs. < HS	1.6**	(1.3 - 2.1)	2.0**	(1.7 - 2.3)
18 - 19 yrs. >= HS	1.2	(0.79 - 1.83)	1.2	(0.97 - 1.49)
>= 20 yrs. < HS	1.1	(0.83 - 1.32)	1.4**	(1.2 - 1.6)
>= 20 yrs. > HS	0.65**	(0.49 - 0.85)	0.86**	(0.76 - 0.96)
Primiparous	0.47**	(0.38 - 0.58)	0.73**	(0.65 - 0.81)
Unmarried	1.6**	(1.3 - 2.1)	1.3**	(1.2 - 1.5)
No Prenatal Care	1.8	(0.96 - 3.38)	2.1**	(1.5 - 3.0)
Inadequate Prenatal Care*	1.3**	(1.1 - 1.6)	1.6**	(1.4 - 1.8)
Intermediate Prenatal Care	0.9	(0.7 - 1.2)	1.0	(0.86 - 1.16)
Adequate+ Prenatal Care	1.3	(0.92 - 1.84)	1.2	(0.98 - 1.47)
Smoking During Pregnancy	1.3	(0.87 - 1.94)	1.6**	(1.4 - 1.7)
Drinking During Pregnancy	1.6**	(1.2 - 2.3)	1.4	(0.9 - 2.1)

* These data were reported previously by the Midwest Maternal and Child Health Data Improvement Project (MMDIP)

** significant at $p <= 0.01$

*** The prenatal care utilization categories used are as defined by the APNCU Index developed by Kotelchuck.

1. Describe the coding for age/education and prenatal care. What are the reference groups? That is, what category for age/education does not appear in the table, and what category of prenatal care does not appear in the table? Do you think these formulations are appropriate?

2. How is parity associated with postneonatal death among low risk infants? Is parity a risk factor or a risk marker?

3. Interpret the meaning of the non-significant odds ratio of 1.1 for black women and the significant one of 1.4 for white women among those who are >= 20 years old with less than a high school education.

4. How adequate is this model for exploring postneonatal mortality among low risk infants? What other variables might be included in a model?

5. Brain teaser. Calculate the odds ratio of the likelihood of a postneonatal death for a woman who is multiparous and unmarried compared to the likelihood of a postneonatal death for a woman who is primiparous and married. All other variables in the model should be held constant. Use the data for white women. (Hint: Write down what the odds ratio would be in terms of the beta coefficients and then from this figure out how to calculate it with the numbers available in the table. So:

$$\text{Odds Ratio}\left(\frac{\text{Multiparous, Unmarried}}{\text{Primiparous, Married}}\right) = \frac{e^?}{e^?}$$

Rates and Percent Distributions

Solution for Exercise A

County	Crude Birth Rate per 1,000 Population	Crude Fertility Rate per 1,000 Females Ages 15-44	% Births to Adolescents	Adolescent Fertility Rate per 1,000 Adolescents Ages 10-17
X	19.8	78.4	4.4	13.6
Y	15.4	49.4	7.6	12.6

County Y has a higher % births to adolescents than County X, but a lower adolescent fertility rate. This is because the adult women in County Y have a lower fertility rate than the adult women in County X resulting in the lower overall birth and fertility rates seen in the above table for County Y. The elevated % births to adolescents in County Y compared to County X, therefore, is due to these differences in the rates for the adult women.

The % births to adolescents is not a rate because adult women who are no longer at risk of delivering in their teen years are included in the denominator. It can be argued that the adolescent fertility rates are a "fairer" comparison of the two counties since they are based solely on the experience of their adolescent populations, unrelated to the experience of other women. On the other hand, some might argue for using % births to adolescents precisely because it reflects the experience of teenage women in relation to the overall fertility behavior in their communities.

Defining excess adolescent fertility must be based on a community standard. It may be that any adolescent childbearing is considered an excess, or this may be determined in relation to a state or national average or goal.

Prevalence vs. Incidence

Solution for Exercise B

1. Students #4, #9, and #16 begin smoking during this time, and ten other students were already smokers and therefore not at risk for becoming smokers, so the incidence rate is 3 / (110-10) or 3.0 %.

2. Nine students were smoking at the time they graduated high school, for a prevalence rate of 9 / 110 or 8.2 %.

3. If smoking behavior among graduating seniors is the same as that for students who dropped out, then the results are good estimates. If smoking status is related to drop out status, then the results may be over or underestimates depending on whether those who finish high school are more or less likely to smoke than those who do not.

Incidence and Prevalence

Solution for Exercise C

1. 50/500 = 10%
2. 65/500 = 13%
3. risk means incidence; # of new cases/population at risk = $\dfrac{15}{450}$ = 3.3%

Incidence and Prevalence

Solution for Exercise D

1. Risk refers to incidence data. Since there is no information about new cases for 1995, this question cannot be answered.

2. 120/1450 = 8.3%

3. 130/1370 = 9.5%

4. No, these two prevalence estimates do not provide any information about the risk of developing asthma among children in Community A.

5. Knowing the incidence rate helps somewhat but does not tell the entire story as children seeking care for their asthma in the ER are not representative of the entire population of children with asthma in Community A. Incidence rate: 42/1282 =3.3%

6. It would be helpful to have baseline information on the incidence rate of childhood asthma diagnoses in the ER at Hospital X in Community A. Short of obtaining information from population based child health surveys over time, it would also be important to obtain data from primary care physicians in the community, other community hospitals, from the schools, and possibly from the pharmacists in the community. In addition, it might be helpful to compare Community A's data to data from similar communities.

Confidence Intervals and Hypothesis Testing
Solution for Exercise E

1.
$$CI = 16.2 \pm 1.96 \sqrt{\frac{16.2}{8,717} \times 1,000} = 16.2 \pm 2.67 = (13.5 - 18.9)$$

$$CI = 13.0 \pm 1.96 \sqrt{\frac{13.0}{5,673} \times 1,000} = 13.0 \pm 2.97 = (10.0 - 16.0)$$

2. Here, "year" is the exposure and "infant death" is the outcome.

		Infant Death	
Year	Yes	No	
1990	141	8,576	8,717
1995	74	5,599	5,673
	215	14,175	14,390

3. The two rates are not statistically different at $p < 0.05$ since Z < the critical value of 1.96. The overall rate to estimate the common variance is 14.9 (215/14,390 x 1,000).

$$z = \frac{(16.2 - 13) - 0}{\sqrt{14.9\left(\frac{1}{8,717} + \frac{1}{5,673}\right) \times 1,000}} = 1.5$$

Confidence Intervals and Hypothesis Testing
Solution for Exercise F

1.
$$CI = 87.3 \pm 1.96 \sqrt{\frac{87.3(100 - 87.3)}{345}} = 87.3 \pm 3.65 = (83.7 - 91.0)$$

$$CI = 79.4 \pm 1.96 \sqrt{\frac{79.4(100 - 79.4)}{726}} = 79.4 \pm 2.94 = (76.5 - 82.3)$$

2.
$$z = \frac{(87.3 - 79.4) - 0}{\sqrt{81.9(100 - 81.9)\left(\frac{1}{345} + \frac{1}{726}\right)}} = 3.14$$

Since 3.14 > 1.96, the two proportions are significantly different at p < 0.05.

3.

$$z = \frac{(87.3 - 90.0) - 0}{\sqrt{\dfrac{90.0(100 - 90.0)}{345}}} = -1.7 \quad \text{and} \quad z = \frac{(79.4 - 90.0) - 0}{\sqrt{\dfrac{90.0(100 - 90.0)}{726}}} = -9.5$$

The immunization status of 2-year-old children in Region 1 is not significantly different from the Year 2000 Objective since -1.7 > -1.96. The immunization status of 2-year-old children in Region 2, however, is significantly below the standard since -9.5 < -1.96.

Preventive Fraction

Solution for Exercise G

1. The incidence of motor vehicle injury among children in car seats is $(20/5,000) \times 10,000 = 40$ per 10,000. The incidence of motor vehicle injury among children not in car seats is $(50/5,000) \times 10,000 = 100$ per 10,000 children.

2. The preventive fraction is 1-relative risk, or 1-(40/100)=0.60. If all of the 5,000 children not using car seats would use them, then $0.60 \times 50 = 30$ injuries in this group could be prevented.

3. The rearranged table is as follows, assuming that the incidence of motor vehicle injury among those children using and not using car seats remains the same:

		Motor Vehicle Injury		
		Yes	No	
Car Seat Use	Yes	30	7,470	7,500
	No	25	2,475	2,500
		55	9,945	10,000

$(30/7,500) \times 10,000 = 40$ per 10,000 children
$(25/2,500) \times 10,000 = 100$ per 10,000 children

And the estimated overall motor vehicle injury rate is reduced from 70 to 55 per 10,000 children.

Ecologic Analysis

Solution for Exercise H

$$\text{Relative Prevalence:} \qquad \frac{0.33}{0.14} = 2.4$$

$$\text{Population Attributable Risk\%:} \qquad \frac{0.20 - 0.14}{0.20} \times 100 = 30\%$$

Counties with limited access to primary care physicians for children have more than twice the risk of being short of the Year 2000 Objective for two-year-old immunization status (RP=2.4). With a PAR% of 30%, the number of counties that might meet the Year 2000 Objective if the supply of primary care physicians were increased to at least 5 per 10,000 children in all of the counties is 0.30 x 10 = 3. In other words, seven rather than ten of the 50 counties would fall short of the Objective.

Multivariable Analysis

Solution for Exercise I

1. Following is output from Epi-Info showing the organization of the 2 × 2 tables, and the measure of association. Payment source is the exposure variable (Medicaid, Non-Medicaid), Disease is either ER admissions or hospital admissions (Yes,No). The relative risks are 2.88 and 2.17 for the crude association between payment source and ER and hospital admissions, respectively. Both associations are statistically significant and have narrow confidence intervals. Children on Medicaid are more than twice as likely as those not on Medicaid to visit the ER or be admitted to the hospital.

```
        CRUDE ASSOCIATIONS

           ER ADMISSIONS
             + Disease -                        Analysis of Single Table
      +--------+--------+                   Odds ratio = 2.92 (2.62 <OR< 3.25)
    +|   990   | 57063  | 58053             Cornfield 95% confidence limits for OR
      +--------+--------+                   Relative risk = 2.88 (2.60 <RR< 3.20)
    -|   540   | 90811  | 91351             Taylor Series 95% confidence limits for RR
      +--------+--------+                   Ignore relative risk if case control study.
    E    1530    147874    149404
    x                                                     Chi-Squares   P-values
    p                                                     -----------   --------
    o                                       Uncorrected  :   434.76     0.0000000 ---
    s                                       Mantel-Haenszel:  434.76    0.0000000 ---
    u                                       Yates corrected:  433.66    0.0000000 ---
    r
    e


        HOSPITAL ADMISSIONS
             + Disease -                        Analysis of Single Table
      +--------+--------+                   Odds ratio = 2.35 (2.26 <OR< 2.43)
    +|  7477   | 50576  | 58053             Cornfield 95% confidence limits for OR
      +--------+--------+                   Relative risk = 2.17 (2.10 <RR< 2.25)
    -|  5416   | 85935  | 91351             Taylor Series 95% confidence limits for RR
      +--------+--------+                   Ignore relative risk if case control study.
    E   12893    136511    149404
    x                                                     Chi-Squares   P-values
    p                                                     -----------   --------
    o                                       Uncorrected  :  2174.96     0.0000000 ---
    s                                       Mantel-Haenszel:  2174.95   0.0000000 ---
    u                                       Yates corrected:  2174.08   0.0000000 ---
    r
    e
```

2. a. Adjusted association is 2.71
    b. Adjusted association is 2.27
    c. While the results of a statistical test for interaction are not available here, the results for each stratum show that County Q has a different, and higher, relative risk for the association between payment source and ER admissions than those for County P and County R (4.72 v. 2.24 and 2.44). For the association between payment source and hospital admissions, the three counties have somewhat different relative risks (1.47, 2.97, and 2.35).
    d. If it is decided that the differences in the stratum specific relative risks constitute effect modification, then confounding is no longer a relevant question. The adjusted or summary measure should not be used as it cannot adequately reflect the stratum specific information. If, on the other hand, it is decided that effect modification is not present, then a comparison of the crude and adjusted relative risks for each association can be made. In this case, it seems useful to report separate county estimates and further investigate the apparent differences.

Two additional variables that could be examined are child age and admission diagnosis. For regression modeling, 2 dummy variables would be created to hold information for the three counties; child age might also be categorized into, say, < 5, 5-14, >14, again requiring 2 dummy variables; admission diagnoses could be grouped and perhaps a continuous severity index created. Logistic regression would be used since the outcome is ER admission (Yes,No), and a model might look like:

ER ADMIT = MEDICAID+COUNTYP+COUNTYQ+LESS5+MORE14+SEVERE

County R is chosen as the reference county and children 5-14 are chosen as the reference age group.

More complicated models with terms for effect modification might also be explored. For example, a variable to examine possible interaction between payment source and severity of diagnosis might be included, calculated as MEDICAID×SEVERE (MEDSEV). The model would then look like:

ER ADMIT = MEDICAID+COUNTYP+COUNTYQ+LESS5+MORE14+SEVERE+MEDSEV

Synthetic Estimation

Solution for Exercise J

Strata	Numbers in County X	State Weighted Proportions	Synthetic Estimate for County X
<= 15, Black	172	0.262	45
<= 15, White	764	0.293	224
16-17, Black	130	0.257	33
16-17, White	681	0.274	187
Total	**1,747**		**489**

1. The stratum specific synthetic estimates of the numbers of high school age youth in County X who would identify themselves as slightly or very overweight appear in the rightmost column of the above table. They are the result of multiplying the state weighted proportions by the numbers in County X. The total of these estimates is 489, yielding a synthetic percentage of 489 / 1,747 or 28.0 %.

2. The synthetic estimate of 28.0 % for County X based on stratification by age and racial designation is not very different from the overall state estimate of 28.4%.

3. The youth in County X are either not very different from those in the State as a whole, in which case the synthetic estimate may be quite accurate, or other stratification variables are needed to yield a more accurate estimate. The MCH professionals in County X need to rely on their knowledge of the demographic and other social, behavioral, and medical characteristics of the youth in the county to assess whether an estimate using these strata is likely to be accurate.

4. Counties might need to work with the state in altering the sampling design of the YRBS to insure that there is enough sample size in strata that the counties think are important if the survey data are to be used to obtain county level estimates.

Interpreting Regression Results

Solution for Exercise K

1. The reference group for age/education includes <u>women >=20 years old with a high school education</u>. This variable differentiates women according to their joint values on age and education. It separates out women ages 18-19 who have appropriately completed high school from their counterparts who have not. It might be useful to further separate women who have completed more than high school into groups for those who have completed college and those who have not. The reference group for prenatal care includes <u>women who received adequate care according to the APNCU Index</u>. The APNCU Index is modified here to distinguish between women with no prenatal care and those who receive inadequate prenatal care.

2. Since the variable is called "primiparous", this indicates that primiparous women are coded "1" and multiparous women are coded "0". With the odds ratio less than 1 for both whites and blacks, it appears that being primiparous is protective for postneonatal death, or conversely that being multiparous is associated with increased likelihood of postneonatal death. Parity may not be a true risk factor, but rather a risk marker, perhaps reflecting differences in the home and/or community of the primiparous and multiparous women. Further investigation is required.

3. The reference group for these odds ratios are women of the same age who have a high school education. The fact that black women with less than a high school education are not shown to be at elevated risk compared to their counterparts with more education, but that white women with less education are at slightly elevated risk compared with their counterparts indicates that educational attainment in our society may have different meaning depending on racial/ethnic characteristics. Assumptions about educational attainment and its relationship to health outcomes must be thought through carefully.

4. This model is not very adequate for examining postneonatal mortality among low risk infants because it does not include variables that can directly assess the social, behavioral, and community factors that may contribute to deaths of infants at low medical risk. Cause specific death information would also refine the analysis.

5. Remember that the beta coefficients from logistic regression are the natural logarithm of the odds ratios. So, the beta coefficient for the variable "primiparous" = ln(0.73)= -0.31, with primiparous women coded "1" and multiparous women coded "0". The beta coefficient for the variable

"unmarried" is ln(1.3) = 0.26, with unmarried women coded "1" and married women coded "0". Therefore:

$$\text{Odds Ratio}\left(\frac{\text{Multiparous, Unmarried}}{\text{Primiparous, Married}}\right) = \frac{e^{-0.31(0)+0.26(1)}}{e^{-0.31(1)+0.26(0)}}$$

$$= e^{-0.3(-1)+0.26(1)}$$

$$= e^{0.57}$$

$$= 1.8$$

References

Bakketeig, L., Hoffman, H., and Oakley, A., "Perinatal Mortality" in *Perinatal Epidemiology*, Eds: Bracken, M., New York: Oxford University Press, 1984, 126.

Campbell, D. and Stanley, J., "Experimental and Quasi-Experimental Designs for Research on Teaching."   In N.L. Gage (Ed.) *Handbook of Research on Teaching.* Chicago: Rand McNally, 1963. Also published as "Experimental and Quasi-Experimental Designs for Research." Chicago: Rand McNally, 1966.

Cook, T. and Campbell, D., *Quasi-Experimentation: Design and Analysis Issues for Field Settings*, Boston: Houghton Mifflin Company, 1979.

Hennekens, C. and Buring, J., *Epidemiology in Medicine,* Boston/Toronto: Little Brown and Company, 1986

Institute of Medicine, *Preventing Low Birthweight.* Washington, D.C.: National Academy Press, 1985.

Levy, P. and Lemeshow, S., *Sampling of Populations: Methods and Applications*, New York: John Wiley Sons, 1991, 33.

Mausner, J. and Kramer, S., *Epidemiology: An Introductory Text, 2nd Edition,* Philadelphia: W.B. Saunders Company, 1985, 155.

Rothman, K., *Modern Epidemiology*, Boston/Toronto: Little Brown and Company, 1986.

Wilcox, Lynne S. and Marks, James S., *From Data to Action: CDC's Public Health Surveillance for Women, Infants and Children*, U.S. Dept. of Health and Human Services, Public Health Service, Centers for Disease Control.

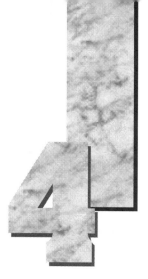

Methods for Summarizing Data

by Deborah Rosenberg, PhD

In public health, multiple population groups, multiple risk factors, and multiple outcomes are often simultaneously of interest. In addition, data analysts must often address the domains of health services and health systems as well as health status. For maternal and child health professionals, census data, vital records data, Medicaid data, hospital discharge data, WIC data, client tracking system data, focus group and other qualitative data, and national and/or local sample survey data are all relevant for describing and monitoring the health of women, infants, children, adolescents, and families. The challenge for MCH data analysts is to summarize this array of data in ways that facilitate carrying out the core functions of assessment, assurance, and policy development.

The process of summarizing data within and across many domains and population groups can seem daunting unless a well defined analysis plan is articulated and implemented. Developing an analysis plan is an essential step in information-based decision making. The aim is to design a systematic approach for reducing the data burden for a given MCH analysis or report. Without such an approach, it is likely that data will not be successfully translated into the information needed by program planners, managers, and policy-makers.

DEVELOPING AN ANALYSIS PLAN

Making analytic choices that result in a cogent portrayal of health status, services, and the relationship between them is as much an art as a science. As a general rule, data are more reliable and easier to interpret as the degree of summarization increases but, conversely, data are more targeted and specific as the degree of summarization decreases. The objective is to weigh the advantages and disadvantages of different strategies and choose the one that strikes the best balance between specificity and interpretability.

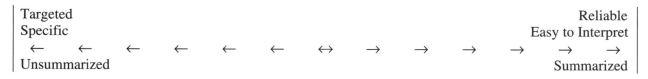

Targeted Specific												Reliable Easy to Interpret
←	←	←	←	←	←	↔	→	→	→	→	→	→
Unsummarized												Summarized

Data summarization strategies can reduce the data burden either directly by limiting the amount of data reported, or indirectly by increasing its interpretability. Often, both approaches are used in combination.

In order for data summarization to be effective, the analysis plan should be framed according to each of the following:

- Purpose of the analysis
- Audience for the analysis
- Data availability and data quality

Each of these is discussed below.

Purpose of the Analysis

Routine surveillance and monitoring, statewide or community based needs assessment, quality assurance activities, program evaluation, and special studies each require development of a distinct analysis strategy. As a starting point, each analysis should be situated within a matrix of pertinent population groups and domains of interest:

Population Groups	Domains		
	Health Status	Health Services	Health Systems
Women			
Infants			
Children			
Adolescents			
Families			

One analysis might be situated in just one cell of the matrix, while another might be situated in all of the cells.

For a comprehensive statewide MCH needs assessment, for example, it is likely that all of the cells of the matrix are appropriate. Many indicators will be of interest as well as comparisons across person, place, time, and risk. In such a wide-ranging analysis, data summarization will be necessary both in terms of restricting the amount of data and using methods that increase interpretability. A certain amount of detail may have to be sacrificed as a safeguard against losing sight of the major findings of the needs assessment.

For community-based needs assessment, all of the cells of the matrix may again be appropriate and many indicators will again be of interest. The data burden, however, will be lighter because the focus is on each area separately rather than on comparisons across areas. Therefore, the degree of data summarization may not have to be as great as for a statewide analysis.

In contrast to needs assessment, intensive study of a particular health problem may situate an analysis in only one cell of the matrix, and only a few indicators will be of interest as well. In this circumstance, it is possible and desirable to disaggregate (leave unsummarized) data for many person, place, time and risk variables. The goal here is to explore one issue in great detail.

For program evaluation, an analysis will, by definition, cross at least the two domains of health status and health services, though often only one population group will be pertinent. Identifying improvement or deterioration in health status over time will be the primary focus, and therefore, data summarization will likely be necessary for other dimensions such as socio-demographic characteristics or geography.

These brief examples illustrate the linkage between data summarization and the purpose of an analysis. You can see that how widely or narrowly the analytic net is cast, whether many or only a few indicators are of interest, and the particular questions being asked, all govern the data summarization process.

The Audience for the Analysis

A particular analysis and report may be intended for use by the professionals working in state or local health agencies; it may be intended for legislators; it may be intended for stakeholders in communities; it may be intended for the general public. The degree and type of data summarization must be matched to the needs of each group. The general public may only need to see statewide figures, whereas legislators may want information stratified by county, and community leaders may want it stratified by even smaller units of geography. One audience may want a comprehensive report, another may want a sound bite. The MCH data analyst should be able to produce quality information for each of these circumstances.

Regardless of the audience, though, the data analyst should always examine the data in its most unsummarized form. If decisions about how much summarization, and on which variables, are made without first looking at the "raw" data, important differences and disparities might be overlooked. For example, a decision might be made to present an indicator for children ages 0-17 stratified by race/ethnicity, when in fact, variation by age is greater than variation across race/ethnic groups. In light of this, a more appropriate data summarization decision would have been to present the data stratified by age and not by race/ethnicity. This would have been clear had the data been examined in their most refined form.

Decisions about how to summarize data, then, should rely less on untested assumptions and more on empirical findings. Depending on the audience, the analyst has to make choices about the degree of summarization, but these choices should be guided by a thorough understanding of the loss of information entailed in each decision.

Availability of Data and Data Quality

Choices about which data to include in an analysis are highly dependent on both the availability of data and on its quality. As MCH professionals, we can all name many indicators that would enhance our ability to carry out the core functions of public health, but for which data are not routinely collected. For example, it would be very informative to report data on the incidence of child injury by type of injury and age. Since incidence data are not readily available, however, hospitalization for injury or injury mortality are typically reported instead, despite the limitations this imposes on our analysis.

Similarly, although it is well accepted that analyzing the content or quality of prenatal care is critical to understanding the effectiveness of this service, generally only measures of the quantity of prenatal care received, such as the timing of the first visit and the total number of visits, are available for inclusion in analysis.

Data quality also limits our analytic choices. For example, gestational age is a critical variable for understanding perinatal morbidity and mortality, but birthweight is more commonly chosen as an indicator because it has been shown to be more accurately documented.

How we summarize data is affected by data availability and data quality. Sometimes we have to present more data than we would like because we need to use several less than optimal measures in an attempt to approximate the information contained in an indicator that is itself unavailable. Sometimes we use data of poor quality because no high quality alternative is available, and perhaps most problematic, sometimes we mis-specify the questions we ask because of the constraints in the data.

Variables, Methods, and Presentation

Framed by the purpose of the analysis, the audience for which it is intended, and the availability and quality of data, the specifics of analysis planning can proceed. The opportunity for data summarization occurs in three successive phases:

Phase I: Selection of variables. This phase includes the selection and definition of the primary indicator or indicators that will be the central focus of the analysis. While the formulation of some MCH indicators, such as the infant mortality rate, are well established, defining numerators and denominators for other indicators is a crucial part of the data summarization process. Similarly, selection and definition of the person, place, time, and risk variables that will be used to refine the analysis of the primary indicator(s) occurs in this phase.

Phase II: Selection of analytic methods. This phase involves decisions about how the indicators and other variables selected will be examined. For example, some indicators might be presented as counts and some as rates; some might be presented as overall averages while others might be stratified by person, place, time, or levels of risk; some indicators might be combined into a composite index; some indicators might be presented in their original form while others might be transformed into categories, ranks, or scores. In addition, comparisons might be made intuitively, or formal statistical testing might be conducted.

Phase III: Selection of presentation format. This phase involves designing a report that effectively communicates the results of the analysis. Written narrative, tables, charts, graphs, and maps are each effective formats depending on the type of data being presented. Organization of each, including defining sections of text, choosing chart types (pie, bar, line, etc.), defining rows and columns for tables, horizontal and vertical (x and y) axes for graphs, and deciding on map layers are important aspects of data summarization.

In the variable selection phase (Phase I), data summarization choices are made to restrict the actual amount of data to be analyzed and reported. The number of indicators can be restricted as well as the number of person, place, time, and risk strata. For instance, from a pool of 50 potential indicators of interest, it might be decided to include only 10 in a given report. Similarly, from a pool of many potential person, place, time, and risk variables, only a few might be selected. The drive to summarize data dictates the exclusion of many variables, and so those that are selected must, if possible, be broadly representative of those that are not.

In the analytic methods phase (Phase II), data summarization choices are made to both restrict the amount of data and to increase its interpretability. Restricting the amount of data is accomplished by limiting the degree of stratification for each of the indicators, drawing from the list of the other selected variables. Possibilities for reporting each indicator might include:

- By age, race/ethnicity, county, and year
- By age, race/ethnicity, and county
- By age, and race/ethnicity
- By age
- Overall for the state for one year

Moving from the most refined to the more summarized levels, a minimal loss of information is assumed (or preferably verified with preliminary analyses). For instance, if you choose to report an indicator without stratifying by county, the assumption is that the indicator does not vary by county in a way that is meaningful, either epidemiologically or from a program or policy perspective.

The aim is to combine only as many strata as necessary to gain reliability in terms of sample size, and ease of interpretation in terms of reducing the amount of data the audience needs to digest. Aggregating across too many strata may obscure meaningful differences, and although the audience will not be overwhelmed, neither will it have useful information. This principle holds whether data will be summarized across person, place, time, or across risk. Over-summarization of socio-demographic characteristics and risk can obscure differences that have implications for program design, and in combination with geography, may have implications for resource allocation. Over-summarization across time can mask patterns of improvement or deterioration, and conceal the impact of critical events such as implementation of new programs or policies.

One strategy for reducing the amount of data reported without sacrificing too much information is to let person, place, time, and risk variables operate jointly. For instance, data can be collapsed in one of these dimensions, and the danger of obscuring meaningful differences minimized if related data from the other dimensions drive the process. To illustrate, if geographic areas are to be combined, some possible approaches are:

- Combine areas according to levels of risk—for example, combine those areas with similar low birthweight rates, or similar childhood immunization rates.

- Combine by socio-demographic factors—for example, combine those areas with similar racial/ethnic composition, similar income, or similar educational levels.

- Combine by level of services/programs in the area—for example, combine those areas with similar numbers of providers per capita, or similar numbers of WIC sites.

Instead of restricting the amount of stratification, another strategy that restricts the amount of data is to report only values that highlight extremes, disparities, or changes. For example, if indicators are being examined by geographic area, only the two areas with the highest rates and the two areas with the lowest rates on each indicator might be reported. Or, only indicators with a three-fold difference across areas might be reported. Attention might be focused on those geographic areas within which there are large disparities between demographically defined population groups. If trends over time are of interest, perhaps only areas that show a 10% improvement or deterioration over time on an indicator might be reported.

Other data summarization techniques used in the methods phase (Phase II) leave the actual amount of data reported unchanged, but reduce the data burden by transforming the data in ways that make it easier for an audience to assimilate. For example, grouping indicator values into discrete categories alleviates the data burden by replacing many distinct values with a few summary ones. Ranking and scoring methods, like categorization, increase the interpretability of data without reducing the amount of data reported. Unlike categorization, though, these methods do not even reduce the number of distinct values, but the ordering and labeling inherent in the transformed values (such as integer ranks) adds information and meaning that the original values could not convey.

Categorization, ranking, and scoring enhance the reader's ability to synthesize information. Care must be taken, however, not to over-use these methods. Report cards, for example, while they are easy to understand, often suffer from over-summarization, yielding a view of a health issue that is too rudimentary to be useful from a program planning or policy perspective.

Index construction is a hybrid of restricting the amount of data and enhancement of data interpretability. It permits two or more indicators to be represented by one composite measure. The number of data values reported is reduced, but rather than excluding indicators from the analysis, the information they contain is merely reflected in a somewhat different form.

In the presentation phase (Phase III), data summarization choices are also made to facilitate interpretability. In general, visual methods such as graphs and maps handle data from many sources and of different types in an integrated and comprehensible form. Suppose, for example, a state has 64 counties. Whereas it may be difficult to scan 64 numbers in a table and make judgements about their relative standing, looking across the heights of bars in a bar chart may be much easier. Text and tables, however, while they may require more effort to absorb, do provide more detailed and specific information.

It is important not to ignore or underestimate the role of text in the data summarization process. Data may have been selected appropriately in Phase I, creative and useful methods applied in Phase II, and effective tables, charts, graphs and maps created to present it in a clear and concise fashion in Phase III, but data summarization is incomplete without explicit narrative interpretation. The data alone cannot fully communicate a message. MCH professionals must take on the responsibility for carrying the data summarization process through to its conclusion by writing text that gives shape to the story that the data only outlines.

The table below reviews the three phases of analysis planning and data summarization:

Summarizing Data: Reducing the Data Burden		
Restricting the Amount of Data	Increasing Interpretability	
Phase I: Variables	Phase II: Methods	Phase III: Presentation

Limit the number of indicators
 	
Limit the number of person, place, time, and risk variables
	Limit the amount of stratification
	
	Transform variables into:
	    Discrete categories
	    Ranks
	    Scores
	
	Construct indices
	
	Use statistical testing
		Text
		
		Tables
		
		Charts
		
		Graphs
		
		Maps

METHODS FOR INCREASING INTERPRETABILITY

Categorization

We saw earlier that categorization can reduce the data burden by condensing many values into a few summary categories. In addition, when multiple indicators are being analyzed, imposing common labels helps to integrate information across the various measures. To illustrate, the first of the two tables below shows the low birthweight rates and child injury mortality rates for 10 counties, and the second of the two tables shows the same data in categorized values. The counties are sorted by the low birthweight rates, and categories are defined as above or below the median on each indicator.

Original Values		
County	Low Birthweight Rate (%)	Child Injury Mortality Rate (per 100,000)
A	4.17	46.60
B	5.68	45.94
C	6.08	47.69
D	6.41	36.55
E	6.49	81.50
F	6.96	31.38
G	7.20	42.83
H	7.75	39.36
I	8.44	30.79
J	21.05	52.64

Summary Categories: Above (+) and Below (-) the Median		
County	Low Birthweight Rate (%)	Child Injury Mortality Rate (per 100,000)
A	-	+
B	-	+
C	-	+
D	-	-
E	-	+
F	+	-
G	+	-
H	+	-
I	+	-
J	+	+

You can see that it is easier to interpret the second table. For example, overall, it does not appear that a high value on one health status indicator necessarily means a high value on the other. Specifically, though, the second table shows that County J is high on both measures while County D is low on both. The distinct values in the first table made it difficult to see this pattern.

In addition to imposing common values, categorizing with intuitive labels is also valuable when the meaning of indicator values is unclear. While some MCH indicators, such as infant mortality, have values that most audiences understand, many indicators do not have values that are so readily interpretable in their original form. For example, many people know without the aid of a label that an infant mortality rate of 15 per 1,000 live births is unacceptably high, but this is not the typical situation. Particularly when there is no standard or goal, such as a national objective, that has been identified and publicized, the meaning of indicator values is not clear. Translating indicator values into intuitive labels such as the following helps the audience find the meaning:

- high, medium, low
- above average, below average
- excellent, good, fair, poor

When possible, a benchmark or external standard, such as a national objective, determines the categorization process. When no such external reference exists, data are categorized according to their relative position in the observed distribution. In "Descriptive Epidemiology and Statistical Estimation", (Module I) we described in some detail various methods for categorizing data, such as defining boundaries such that there are equal numbers of observations in each category or such that there are equal portions of the range of values in each category; we also demonstrated that natural breakpoints or clustering in the data may define category boundaries, and that statistics such as the mean, median, or standard deviation may be used as well.

In the above table (previous page), the median of the observed values was used to define two categories for the 10 low birthweight rates and child injury mortality rates. Following are two approaches to assigning the 10 county low birthweight rates to four categories. As you look at the data again, notice the extreme gap between the highest rate of 21.05 in County J and the next highest rate of 8.44 in County I. Also notice that only County A with its low birthweight rate of 4.17 has met the Year 2000 Objective of 5 low birthweight births in every 100 live births.

2 Possible Ways to Categorize 10 Low Birthweight Rates				
	Method I		Method II	
Category	County	Rate (%)	County	Rate (%)
1	A	4.17	A	4.17
	B	5.68		
			B	5.68
	C	6.08	C	6.08
2	D	6.41	D	6.41
	E	6.49	E	6.49
	F	6.96	F	6.96
3	G	7.20	G	7.20
	H	7.75	H	7.75
			I	8.44
	I	8.44		
4	J	21.05	J	21.05

To the extent possible, Method I divides the 10 observations equally into the four categories. This results in the rates of 8.44 and 21.05 being in the same group, a questionable approach. Method II uses the Year 2000 Objective of 5 % low birthweight births to define the boundary between categories 1 and 2, and also isolates the highest rate of 21.05 because of its extreme value.

Regardless of the chosen breakpoints, defining discrete categories results in loss of information. The values 1-4 cannot possibly be as descriptive as the ten original values for each county.

In either method, for example, the rates of 6.08, 6.41 and 6.49 in Counties C, D and E are grouped together, implying that they are the same. Assessment of an acceptable loss of detail should determine the number of categories to use for a particular indicator; as we've already seen, loss of information can be offset by the gain in interpretability that categorization provides.

Comment

The level of the data will influence the choice of how to define discrete categories. Categorizing a set of birthweight values for individual infants, for example, will require a different strategy than categorizing a set of aggregate low birthweight rates for counties such as that shown in the above examples. For individual level birthweight data, the clinically relevant categories of very low birthweight (< 1500 grams), moderately low birthweight (1500-2499 grams), and "normal" birthweight (>= 2500 grams) are typically used.

Question: Below are the sorted values of the child injury mortality rates for the 10 counties. The overall child injury mortality rate for the 10 counties combined is 42.77 per 100,000 children. Describe a possible categorization strategy.

County	Child Injury Mortality Rate (per 100,000)
I	30.79
F	31.38
D	36.55
H	39.36
G	42.83
B	45.94
A	46.60
C	47.69
J	52.64
E	81.50

Answer: There are many possible categorization strategies for this indicator. One might be as follows:

Category	County	Child Injury Mortality Rate (per 100,000)
1	I	30.79
	F	31.38
2	D	36.55
	H	39.36
3	G	42.83
	B	45.94
	A	46.60
	C	47.69
4	J	52.64
5	E	81.50

This strategy highlights both low and high rates, including emphasizing the potential significance of the two highest rates of 52.64 and 81.50. The overall rate of 42.77 is used to define the breakpoint between the two middle categories.

While the common labels that discrete categories impose, such as "high" and "low", increase the comparability across indicators, they do so in a fairly crude fashion. A more refined transformation is required if precise comparisons are desired. Here again are the low birthweight rate and the child injury mortality rate for County J along with the median on each indicator for the 10 counties:

	Low Birthweight Rate (%)	Child Injury Mortality Rate (per 100,000)
County J	21.05	52.64
Median of the 10 Counties	6.73	44.38

Earlier we saw that both of County J's rates were labeled "+", indicating that each was above its respective median, but although we know they are both high, it is impossible to judge which of County J's indicators is actually "farther" from the median. Is a 14 % difference (21.05 v. 6.73) better or worse than a 8 per 100,000 difference (52.64 v. 44.38)?

It is difficult to achieve precision with a few discrete categories, and therefore, it may be preferable to transform the original values to a common metric or scale using ordinal or continuous (uncategorized) measures such as integer ranks or z-scores. These methods transform the original values such that there is little or no loss of information—the same number of values exist after the transformation as existed before. For example, the 10 indicator values for the 10 counties can be transformed into 10 ranks or 10 z-scores.

Whereas a category label such as "high" or "+" might have a somewhat different meaning from one indicator to the next, an integer rank such as "1" or a score such as "1.3" will have the same meaning across indicators. Some ranking and scoring methods are described below.

Integer Ranking

Simple ranking assigns integers to the sorted values of the indicator of interest. For instance, if 10 counties are to be ranked according to the percent of children living in poverty, the integers 1 through 10 would be assigned. By definition, the differences between the ranks are uniform: the distance between rank 2 and rank 4 is equal to the distance between all other values that are two ranks apart.

Integer ranking can be applied to individual or aggregate level data, although it is most often used for aggregate values. Here are the 10 county low birthweight rates transformed into 10 integer ranks:

Integer Ranking of 10 Low Birthweight Rates		
County	%	Rank
A	4.17	1
B	5.68	2
C	6.08	3
D	6.41	4
E	6.49	5
F	6.96	6
G	7.20	7
H	7.75	8
I	8.44	9
J	21.05	10

Continuous scoring methods such as percentile rescaling, z-scores, and z-tests also assign ordered values to the original data, but unlike integer ranking these values are not uniformly spaced. Instead, scoring methods assign new values that preserve the original distribution of the data, leaving the relative distances between values unchanged.

Percentile Rescaling

The goal of percentile rescaling is to translate the position of a value on one scale to exactly the same position on another. For example, this approach will translate a value at the 25th percentile along the original distribution of values, and find a value at the 25th percentile along a new range. This transformation can be accomplished in two steps:

First, let's examine the formula for finding the percentile of a known value:

$$\text{Percentile} = \frac{\text{Original Value} - \text{Lowest Original Value}}{\text{Highest Original Value} - \text{Lowest Original Value}} \times 100$$

The numerator in this equation is a measure of how far along the original range a given value is—its distance from the lowest value on this range. The denominator is a measure of the entire original range—the distance from the lowest to the highest value. The ratio of these two, then, is the percentile of the value of interest.

Returning to the example of the 10 county low birthweight rates, remember that the range was from the lowest rate of 4.17% in County A to the highest rate of 21.05% in County J. Let's consider County C's rate of 6.08 and determine its position along this range. All of the terms on the right-hand side of the equation are known, and we solve for the unknown percentile:
:

$$\text{Percentile} = \frac{6.08 - 4.17}{21.05 - 4.17} \times 100$$

$$= \frac{1.91}{16.88} \times 100$$

$$= 11.3$$

County C's rate of 6.08 is a distance of 1.91 beyond the lowest value of 4.17, and 1.91 is 11.3% along the whole range of 16.88.

Second, to place 6.08 on a scale with a minimum value of 1 and a maximum value of 10, for example, we need to find the value located at 11.3% along this new range. The calculation is set up the same as before except that the equation is now written in terms of the new values rather than the original ones:

$$\text{Percentile} = \frac{\text{New Value} - \text{Lowest New Value}}{\text{Highest New Value} - \text{Lowest New Value}} \times 100$$

This time, the value of the percentile is known, along with the highest and lowest values of the new range, and we solve for the unknown new value. For County C's low birthweight rate, we have:

$$11.3 = \frac{\text{New Value} - 1}{10 - 1} \times 100$$

Then, the equation is algebraically reorganized to solve for the new value:

$$\text{New Value} = \frac{(10 - 1) \times 11.3}{100} + 1$$

$$= \frac{9 \times 11.3}{100} + 1$$

$$= 2.02$$

This new value of 2.02 is at exactly the same point along the range of 1 to 10, as is the original value of 6.08 along the range of 4.17 to 21.05, as is 11.3 along the range of 0 to 100. Similarly, the values of 5.5, 12.61, and 50 are at the same point (50th percentile). The equivalence across the three ranges is illustrated below:

Equivalent Values on Three Different Scales

	*		
1.00	2.02	5.5	10.00

	*		
4.17	6.08	12.61	21.05

	*		
0.00	11.30	50	100.00

Here are the results of applying the percentile rescaling process to all 10 of the county low birthweight rates :

Integer Ranking and Percentile Rescaling of 10 Low Birthweight Rates			
County	Original Values (%)	Rank	New Scale 1-10
A	4.17	1	1.00
B	5.68	2	1.80
C	6.08	3	2.02
D	6.41	4	2.19
E	6.49	5	2.24
F	6.96	6	2.49
G	7.20	7	2.62
H	7.75	8	2.91
I	8.44	9	3.28
J	21.05	10	10.00

You can see that the percentile rescaled values are in the same order as the values of the original data. Unlike simple integer ranking, however, the distances between values are not uniform; the distances between the rescaled values mirror their relative distances in the original data. For example, in the above table, the distance between the integer ranks for Counties B and D is, of course, 2 (4-2), while the distance between the rescaled values for these two counties is only 0.39 (2.19-1.80). Conversely, the percentile rescaling is able to preserve the extreme gap between the highest rate of 21.05 and the next highest of 8.44 with a distance of 6.72 (10.0-3.28), while the integer rank difference is only 1 (10-9).

With percentile rescaling, a common range is chosen for all indicators. In the example for the 10 county data, the lowest value (at 0% along the range) of any indicator would be assigned the new value of "1" and the highest value (at 100% along the range) of any indicator would be assigned a new value of "10". All of the intermediate values would likewise be assigned equivalent values—a value at the 11.3th percentile *on any indicator* would be assigned a new value of 2.02 as was the low birthweight rate for County C.

This form of rescaling can be applied to individual or aggregate level data, although it is typically used with aggregate values.

Comment and Example

The rescaling process can be carried out in just one step, by solving the equations for the original values and the new values simultaneously as follows:

$$\frac{\text{New Value} - \text{New Low}}{\text{New High} - \text{New Low}} = \frac{\text{Original Value} - \text{Original Low}}{\text{Original High} - \text{Original Low}}$$

$$\text{New Value} - \text{New Low} = \frac{\text{Original Value} - \text{Original Low}}{\text{Original High} - \text{Original Low}} \times \text{New High} - \text{New Low}$$

$$\text{New Value} = \left(\frac{\text{Original Value} - \text{Original Low}}{\text{Original High} - \text{Original Low}} \times \text{New High} - \text{New Low} \right) + \text{New Low}$$

In this formulation, County C's low birthweight rate is rescaled as follows:

County C

$$\frac{\text{New Value} - 1}{10 - 1} = \frac{6.08 - 4.17}{21.05 - 4.17}$$

$$\text{New Value} - 1 = \frac{1.91}{16.88} \times 9$$

$$\text{New Value} = (0.113 \times 9) + 1$$

$$= 2.02$$

Consider a few additional examples of using this formulation, beginning with the two endpoints of the range—County A and County J with low birthweight rates of 4.17 and 21.05 respectively:

County A   County J

$$\frac{\text{New Value} - 1}{10 - 1} = \frac{4.17 - 4.17}{21.05 - 4.17} \qquad \frac{\text{New Value} - 1}{10 - 1} = \frac{21.05 - 4.17}{21.05 - 4.17}$$

$$\text{New Value} - 1 = \frac{0}{16.88} \times 9 \qquad \text{New Value} - 1 = \frac{16.88}{16.88} \times 9$$

$$\text{New Value} = (0 \times 9) + 1 \qquad \text{New Value} = (1 \times 9) + 1$$

$$= 1 \qquad\qquad\qquad = 10$$

And, here is percentile rescaled value for County H with a low birthweight rate of 7.75:

County H

$$\frac{\text{New Value} - 1}{10 - 1} = \frac{7.75 - 4.17}{21.05 - 4.17}$$

$$\text{New Value} - 1 = \frac{3.58}{16.88} \times 9$$

$$\text{New Value} = (0.212 \times 9) + 1$$

$$= 2.91$$

Question: For the 10 county data, transform County C's child injury mortality rate of 47.69 to its equivalent percentile position on a scale of 1-10.

Answer: The rescaled value for County C's child injury mortality rate is as follows:

County C

$$\frac{\text{New Value} - 1}{10 - 1} = \frac{47.69 - 30.79}{81.50 - 30.79}$$

$$\text{New Value} - 1 = \frac{16.90}{50.71} \times 9$$

$$\text{New Value} = (0.333 \times 9) + 1$$

$$= 4.00$$

Question: Compare the percentile rescaling results for County C's low birthweight rate and child injury mortality rate with the results from using the categories above and below the median, and integer ranking.

Answer: Here are the results for County C using the three methods discussed so far:

County C	Low Birthweight Rate = 6.08 %	Child Injury Mortality Rate = 47.69 per 100,000
Above (+) and Below (-) the Median	-	+
Integer Ranks	3	8
Percentile Rescaled Values	2.02	4.00

County C's low birthweight rate is below the median of the 10 counties while its child injury mortality rate is above the median of the 10 counties. This dichotomous categorization gives the impression that County C is doing well with regard to low birthweight, but poorly with regard to child injury mortality. The disparate integer ranks of 3 and 8 give the same impression. In contrast, because of the relative distribution of the 10 counties on each indicator, the percentile rescaled values of 2.02 and 4.00 are closer together, both less than half the distance along the range of 1 to 10.

Z-Scores

The classic method for "standardizing" a set of values (finding a common metric or scale) is calculation of z-scores. Instead of translating data to a fixed range as with percentile rescaling, z-scores are anchored by the mean and standard deviation of the original values, and rescaled such that the new mean is 0 and the new standard deviation is 1. The resulting z-scores correspond to points on the standard normal curve, with a theoretical range of approximately -3 to +3. The actual range for each indicator, however, will be different.

Z-scores can be calculated for individual level or aggregate level data. In either case, each value is treated as an "individual" member of a sample. The sample size, then, is equal to the total number of "individuals". When z-scores are calculated for aggregate data, such as county rates and percents, the county is the "individual" (unit of analysis), the group of counties is the sample, and the sample size is therefore the total number of counties. The formula for calculating z-scores is as follows:

Individual Level Data

$$z_i = \frac{X_i - \overline{X}}{\sqrt{\dfrac{\sum_{i-1}^{n}(X_i - \overline{X})^2}{n-1}}}$$

where X_i = the original value
for individual i

and $\overline{X}$ = the mean of the distribution
of individuals

and n = the total number
of individuals

Aggregate Level Data

$$z_i = \frac{p_i - \overline{p}}{\sqrt{\dfrac{\sum_{i=1}^{n}(p_i - \overline{p})^2}{(n-1)}}}$$

where p_i = the original proportion
for county i (or region, census tract, etc.)

and $\overline{p}$ = the mean of the distribution
of counties (or regions, census tracts, etc.)

and n = the total number
of counties (or regions, census tracts, etc.)

For the 10 county data, the mean of the 10 low birthweight rates is:

$$\frac{4.17 + 5.68 + 6.08 + 6.41 + 6.49 + 6.96 + 7.20 + 7.75 + 8.44 + 21.05}{10} = 8.02$$

And the standard deviation is:

$$\sqrt{\frac{(4.17 - 8.02)^2 + (5.68 - 8.02)^2 + K + (8.44 - 8.02)^2 + (21.05 - 8.02)^2}{9}} = 4.72$$

Therefore, the z-score for County C's low birthweight rate is:

$$z_C = \frac{6.08 - 8.02}{4.72} = -0.41$$

And, the z-score for County H's low birthweight rate is:

$$z_H = \frac{7.75 - 8.02}{4.72} = -0.06$$

Here are the results of calculating z-scores for all 10 of the county low birthweight rates :

Integer Ranking and z-score for all of the county low birthweight rates:			
County	Original Values (%)	Rank	z-score
A	4.17	1	-0.82
B	5.68	2	-0.50
C	6.08	3	-0.41
D	6.41	4	-0.34
E	6.49	5	-0.32
F	6.96	6	-0.23
G	7.20	7	-0.17
H	7.75	8	-0.06
I	8.44	9	0.09
J	21.05	10	2.76

Like integer ranking and percentile rescaling, the z-scores are in the same order as the values in the original data. The distances between z-scores are also not uniform, but mirror the relative distances between the original values. The distance between the z-scores for counties B and D is 0.16 (-0.34--0.50) compared to the integer rank difference of 2 (4-2). And, the distance between the z-scores for Counties I and J is 2.67 (2.76–0.09) compared to the integer rank difference of 1 (10-9).

Different than percentile rescaling, z-scores not only maintain the relative distances between values *within* each indicator, they also maintain relative differences *across* indicators. Using the varying standard deviations rather than a fixed range, values at the same percentile will have different z-scores if the standard deviations of the indicators are not equivalent. Generally, z-scores should not be interpreted as tests of statistical significance. Being anchored by the mean of the distribution, though, they can identify values as above or below average—negative versus positive scores. If the distribution is skewed, however, these negative and positive scores may be misleading. Notice that the distribution of the 10 county low birthweight rates is indeed skewed. Because of County J's extreme rate of 21.05 %, the mean of 8.02 used in calculating the z-scores is not a very good measure of the center of the distribution. Recall that in a normal distribution, the values of the mean and the median are the same, but we saw earlier that the median of the low birthweight rates is 6.73, far below this mean of 8.02. As a result, only Counties I and J have positive z-scores (scores higher than the mean), while the eight other counties have negative ones (scores lower than the mean).

Comment and Example

The coefficient of variation (CV), or the ratio of the standard deviation to the mean, measures the relative variability in a set of values. The larger the CV, the wider the range of z-scores. A value at the same percentile of two distributions will have a larger z-score if its distribution has a larger CV than the other distribution. To illustrate, the mean of the low birthweight rates for the 10 counties, as we've seen, is 8.02% and the standard deviation is 4.72; the mean of the child injury mortality rates is 45.52 per 100,000 children and the standard deviation is 14.5. The low birthweight rates have a larger CV than do the child injury mortality rates:

$$CV = \frac{\text{Standard Deviation}}{\text{Mean}}$$

$$\frac{4.72}{8.02} = 0.59 > \frac{14.5}{45.52} = 0.32$$

Therefore, the z-score for a low birthweight rate at a given percentile along the range of low birthweight rates will be larger than the z-score for a child injury mortality rate at the same percentile along the range of child injury mortality rates.

Question: For the 10 county data, calculate a z-score for County C's child injury mortality rate of 47.69. The mean of the 10 county rates is 45.52 and the standard deviation is 14.50.

Answer: The z-score for County C's child injury mortality rate is as follows:

$$z_C = \frac{47.69 - 45.52}{14.50} = 0.15$$

Question: Compare the z-scores for County C's low birthweight rate and child injury mortality rate with the results of percentile rescaling, the categories above and below the median, and integer ranking.

Answer: Here are the results for County C using the four methods discussed so far:

County C	Low Birthweight Rate = 6.08 %	Child Injury Mortality Rate = 47.69 per 100,000
Above (+) and Below (-) the Median	-	+
Integer Ranks	3	8
Percentile Rescaled Values	2.02	4.00
z-scores	-0.41	0.15

We described earlier how the percentile rescaled values for the two indicators were more similar than either the integer ranks or the dichotomous categories, although all three methods indicate that County C's child injury mortality rate is relatively "worse" than its low birthweight rate. The z-score of -0.41 for low birthweight is below its mean while the one of 0.15 for child injury mortality is above its mean, indicating the same pattern as in the other methods. Both measures, though, are less than one standard deviation away from their respective means, implying that the difference between them is not great.

Z-Tests

Z-tests are designed to test hypotheses about summary statistics and therefore, by definition, they are only applied to aggregate level data. In "Measures of Association and Hypothesis Testing", we described z-tests in some detail, both for comparing two independent proportions or rates, or for comparing a proportion or rate to a standard. In the context of data summarization, z-tests may be used to increase the interpretability of data by comparing an entire set of values to a common standard; identifying statistical significance is of secondary importance. Different than z-scores, z-tests do not assume that a set of aggregate values are "individual" members of the same sample; instead, each aggregate value is properly considered a summary of values from a distinct sample with its own distribution. The sample size, then, varies according to the number of individuals at risk in each sample.

A set of z-tests is in a sense a set of "weighted" z-scores since the z value assigned to a given county, for example, is "weighted" by the number of individuals at risk in that county. The varying reliability of the rates in different counties is thus taken into account. The "scores" are the results of the separate statistical tests of the difference between each county indicator and a standard; they are not points on one curve. The standard used may be the overall or weighted mean of the observed data, or an external standard such as observed data from a state or the nation, or a state or national goal.

The formula for calculating z-tests is as follows:

$$\text{Binomial (percents)} \qquad\qquad \text{Poisson (rates)}$$

$$z_i = \frac{p_i - \overline{p}_{tot}}{\sqrt{\dfrac{\overline{p}_{tot}(100 - \overline{p}_{tot})}{n_i}}} \qquad\qquad z_i = \frac{r_i - \overline{r}_{tot}}{\sqrt{\dfrac{\overline{r}_{tot}(*)}{n_i}}}$$

where p_i or r_i = the indicator for county i

and $\overline{p}_{tot}$ or $\overline{r}_{tot}$ = either the overall (weighted) indicator
for all counties combined, or a "standard"

and n_i = the total number of individuals at risk in County i

and $* = 1, 100, 1,000, K, 100,000$, etc.,
according to the units in the denominator

For the 10 county data, the overall low birthweight rate (weighted mean) is:

$$\frac{14 + 193 + 41 + 129 + 12 + 38 + 124 + 93 + 59 + 24}{336 + 3397 + 674 + 2013 + 185 + 546 + 1723 + 1200 + 699 + 114} \times 100$$

$$= \frac{727}{10887} \times 100$$

$$= 6.68$$

The numerator is the sum of the low birthweight births in each county, and the denominator is the sum of the total live births in each county.

The z-test for County C, then, is:

$$z_C = \frac{6.08 - 6.68}{\sqrt{\dfrac{6.68(100 - 6.68)}{674}}}$$

$$= -0.62$$

And, the z-test for County H is:

$$z_H = \frac{7.75 - 6.68}{\sqrt{\dfrac{6.68(100 - 6.68)}{1200}}}$$

$$= 1.48$$

Here are the results of calculating z-tests for all 10 of the county low birthweight rates :

County	Number of Live Births	Original Values (%)	Rank	z-tests
	Integer Ranking and z-tests for 10 County Low Birthweight Rates			
A	336	4.17	1	-1.84
B	3397	5.68	2	-2.33
C	674	6.08	3	-0.62
D	2013	6.41	4	-0.48
E	185	6.49	5	-0.10
F	546	6.96	6	0.26
G	1723	7.20	7	0.87
H	1200	7.75	8	1.49
I	699	8.44	9	1.87
J	114	21.05	10	6.15

Unlike integer ranking, rescaling with percentiles, or z-scores, z-tests do not necessarily correspond to the order in the original data; adjusting for the varying population sizes may alter the ordering. You can see that the z-tests for Counties A and B are not in the same order as their original values or the integer ranks shown above. This is because the relatively large number of live births in County B added "weight" to its score. For z-tests, then, the distance between scores is a function of both the distances in the original data and of the varying population sizes.

Even when population sizes are essentially equal, z-scores and z-tests will be slightly different because of the differing assumptions underlying each method and the resulting differences in the calculational methods used. Remember that z-scores treat aggregate values as though they were values for individuals; z-tests, on the other hand, treat aggregate values as statistics that summarize distinct samples of values for individuals.

Weighted by the varying population sizes in the 10 counties, the overall mean of 6.68 used to calculate the z-tests for the low birthweight rates is a better measure of the center of the distribution than the unweighted mean of 8.02 used earlier in the calculation of z-scores. This value is very close to 6.73, the median of the distribution, and therefore, five of the counties (A-E) have negative z-tests and the other five (F-J) have positive ones.

Because z-tests treat each aggregate value separately, z-tests do not result in a truly common metric across indicators. The ranges in scores can be quite different for different indicators. One indicator may measure the occurrence of a fairly common health event, another may measure the occurrence of a rare event. The z-tests are sensitive to these differences.

Further, one indicator may be based on all live births, another on children < 18 years old, another on the total population. The z-tests are also sensitive to the differences in size of these denominators just as they are sensitive to the differences in the size of populations across geographic areas. The more common the health event and the larger the denominator, the larger the z-test result will be.

Comment and Example

Here are the z-tests for 2 indicators, one measured per 100 (common), the other per 1,000 (rare), each compared to a standard of 9 (per 100 or per 1,000), and each based on a population at risk of 500.

Relatively Rare Event
Relatively Small Population

$$z = \frac{12 - 9}{\sqrt{\frac{9}{500} \times 1,000}}$$

$$= 0.71$$

Relatively Rare Event
Relatively Large Population

$$z = \frac{12 - 9}{\sqrt{\frac{9}{1,000} \times 1,000}}$$

$$= 1.00$$

Now, here are the z-tests for 2 indicators, both measured per 100, each compared to a standard of 9 per 100, one based on a population at risk of 500, and the other on a population at risk of 1,000.

Relatively Common Event
Relatively Small Population

$$z = \frac{12 - 9}{\sqrt{\frac{9(100 - 9)}{500}}}$$

$$= 2.34$$

Relatively Common Event
Relatively Large Population

$$z = \frac{12 - 9}{\sqrt{\frac{9(100 - 9)}{1,000}}}$$

$$= 3.31$$

Notice that the smallest of the four z-tests is that of 0.71 for the rare event measured in a small population; the largest of the z-tests is that of 3.31 for a common event measured in a large population.

Thus far, all of the scoring methods discussed have assigned values according to some internal feature of the observed data, either the median, the range, the unweighted or weighted mean, and/or the standard deviation. One advantage of using z-tests is that they can be anchored to an external standard, which is independent of the distribution of the observed data. Scoring with measures internal to the observed data can only tell us how a particular area is doing in comparison to the other areas being analyzed; the overall standing of all of the areas is not considered. For instance, a county's rate may be two standard deviations "worse" than the mean rate of all of the counties, but this score has quite a different public health meaning depending on whether all of the counties have already met or surpassed an objective for this indicator, some of the counties have met or surpassed the objective while others have not, or none of the counties has yet met or surpassed the objective. An example of this issue is depicted in the graph below:

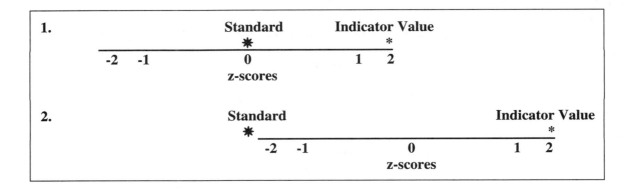

For indicator #1, approximately half of the counties have already met the standard while the other half have not; for indicator #2, none of the counties has yet met the standard. Reporting a z-score of 2 for both indicators for the one county obscures this important difference. Similarly, having a negative z-score has a very different interpretation depending on the indicator; for indicator #1, counties with negative z-scores have met the standard, but for indicator #2, counties with negative z-scores have not met the standard.

Use of an external standard also provides a reference over time. For example, a county may have a z-score of 2 in comparison to other counties for five successive years, but along with the other counties, it may be making progress toward an objective, as measured by improving z-tests of 2.0, 1.5, and 1.0 over the same five year period. The z-tests anchored to an external standard, then, tell a different and important story.

Our discussion of z-tests has focused on their merits from an analytic and statistical perspective, but it must be acknowledged that accounting for varying population size is not always viewed as an advantage by public health professionals or other stakeholders. If 2 counties have exactly the same rate on a health indicator, but very different population sizes, their integer ranks, percentile rescaled values, and z-scores will also be identical, but their z-tests will be different. The question is always raised, "If our rate and their rate is the same, why do we have a worse score?"

Suppose, for example, that in one year, two counties each have an infant mortality rate of 9 infant deaths per 1,000 live births. This rate might hypothetically be ranked 25th out of 50 counties, might be at the 50th percentile, and have a z-score of 0. Now further suppose that one county is rural with very few live births each year, while the other is urban with many live births each year. The z-test for the rural county may not indicate that its rate is statistically different than a standard ($z <= 1.96$, $p >= 0.05$), but the z-test for the urban county may show a significant result for the same rate ($z > 1.96$, $p < 0.05$).

Some would argue that it is unfair to imply by way of these varying z-tests that the urban county is doing worse than the rural one when in fact their rates are identical. We have more confidence, however, in the accuracy of the rate observed in the urban county since it is based on a large sample size, whereas the accuracy of the rate in the rural county is in question since it is based on a small sample size. In fact, having a "worse" z-test despite identical rates could be used as evidence of the need for additional resources.

It should be noted that z-tests do not always show areas with large populations to be "worse" than their less populated counterparts; if two areas, one large and one small, have both met a standard, the z-test for the large area will imply that it is doing better than the small area even if their rates are the same; in other words, a z-test for a large area will always be farther away from zero than a z-test for a small area with the same rate, whether the values are in the positive or negative direction.

Summary of Categorization / Ranking / Scoring Methods

Discrete Categories	Some loss of information—many distinct values are condensed into only a few. Reduces the number of values an audience has to assimilate: easy to interpret if labels are intuitive such as "high" and "low".
Integer Ranking	Preserves the order of the sorted data as well as the number of values, but imposes a uniform set of distances between data points. Audiences can readily understand the meaning of being ranked "1st", "5th", "50th", "100th", etc.
Percentile Rescaling	Preserves the order of the sorted data, the number of values, and the relative distances between data points. A given percentile on any range of original values will be assigned the same position on the new common range. The new range can be for example, 1 to 10, 1 to 100, 0 to 5, -5 to +5.
z-scores	Preserves both the order of the sorted data and the relative distances between data points, and also accounts for differing variability across indicators. By definition, yields a center of 0, but the scores are somewhat less readily understood by general audiences.
z-tests	Both the order of the data and the relative distances between the data points are "adjusted" according to the varying population sizes in the areas of interest. Also sensitive to how common or rare the health event being measured; does not result in a truly common metric across indicators, although values and ranges are usually similar. The value of the scores is determined by the value used as the "standard"; an external standard adds equivalence across indicators and within an indicator over time.

Question: For the 10 county data, calculate a z-test for County C's child injury mortality rate of 47.69 per 100,000. The overall mean of the 10 county data is 42.77 and the population of children < 18 in County C is 13,480.

Answer: The z-test for County C's child injury mortality rate is as follows:

$$z_C = \frac{47.69 - 42.77}{\sqrt{\dfrac{42.77}{13,480} \times 100,000}} = -0.28$$

Question: Compare the z-tests for County C's low birthweight rate and child injury mortality rate with the z-scores, the results of percentile rescaling, the categories above and below the median, and integer ranking.

Answer: Here are the results for County C using five methods:

County C	Low Birthweight Rate = 6.08 %	Child Injury Mortality Rate = 47.69 per 100,000
Above (+) and Below (-) the Median	-	+
Integer Ranks	3	8
Percentile Rescaled Values	2.02	4.00
z-scores	-0.41	0.15
z-tests	-0.62	0.28

The z-tests, as with the other methods, show that County C's low birthweight rate is lower than its child injury mortality rate, in comparison to the other nine counties. The dichotomous categories and the integer ranks imply that this difference is quite large; the percentile rescaled values, z-scores, and z-tests imply it is quite small. The z-tests, however, do imply a somewhat larger difference than do the z-scores— -0.62-0.28 is greater than -0.41-0.15 —because of the assumptions of the method and because low birthweight is a much more common event than child injury mortality.

Index Construction

In the broadest terms, an index is any measure that expresses relative values of a phenomenon. Any single ordinal or continuous variable meets this definition; the infant mortality rate, for example, can be considered an "index" of infant death.

More commonly, though, the term index implies that information from more than one data element has been combined into one composite measure. In addition, an index is usually meant to be used over time, and therefore, comparison to a standard that is fixed over time should be built in to maximize its effectiveness.

There are many different types of indices. An index may be based on either individual or aggregate level data, and may combine variables which are related to the same indicator, may combine variables which cross distinct indicators, but which are related to a larger construct, or may combine variables which cross constructs, but which are related as dimensions of a larger, complex system. Below are a few brief examples illustrating various types of indices.

1.   Combining variables which are related to the same indicator.

An index of low birthweight might combine both the numbers of low birthweight births with the low birthweight rate (%) in order to simultaneously address the service burden and the rate of occurrence. Both a high number of low birthweight births and a high rate will be considered indicative of a problem. Here are the results for all 10 counties using integer ranks:

County	Integer Ranks for Number of Low Birthweight Births		Integer Ranks for Low Birthweight Rate (%)		Index Scores of Low Birthweight Mean of the 2 Ranks
A	2	(14)	1	(4.17)	1.5
B	10	(193)	2	(5.68)	6.0
C	5	(41)	3	(6.08)	4.0
D	9	(129)	4	(6.41)	6.5
E	1	(12)	5	(6.49)	3.0
F	4	(38)	6	(6.96)	5.0
G	8	(124)	7	(7.20)	7.5
H	7	(93)	8	(7.75)	7.5
I	6	(60)	9	(8.44)	7.5
J	3	(24)	10	(21.05)	6.5

Considering the number of low birthweight births along with the low birthweight rate draws a different picture than when the low birthweight rate was considered alone. Counties G, H, and County I, rather than County J have the highest index score (7.5 v. 6.5), and County D, although ranked only fourth in terms of its low birthweight rate, is tied with County J on the composite index.

Another index of low birthweight might consider the current low birthweight % in combination with the trend in the rate over the past several years of data. One possible set of categories could be created as follows:

1. Low birthweight rate below the median and rate decreasing
2. Low birthweight rate above the median and rate decreasing
3. Low birthweight rate below the median and rate constant or increasing
4. Low birthweight rate above the median and rate constant or increasing

Notice that the index scores are ordered such that category 1 is the "best" and category 4 is the "worst". In addition, the *trend* in the low birthweight rate takes precedence over the current level of the rate; counties with low birthweight rates below the median but which show deterioration or no improvement over time are assigned a worse score (3) than counties with low birthweight rates above the median but which show improvement over time which are assigned a better score (2). In other words, a constant or increasing rate is considered a more powerful marker of a problem than the current level of the rate itself.

There are many alternative ways to choose the number of categories and the ordering of the categories for an index. Using the mean of the integer ranks for the number of low birthweight births and the rate of low birthweight resulted in an index with 10 categories for the 10 counties, whereas using above and below the median and decreasing and increasing trends in low birthweight resulted in a four category index. Also, in the four category approach, the ordering of the categories might have given precedence to the current level of the rate rather than the trend in the rate—categories 2 and 3 could be reversed.

2. Combining variables which cross distinct indicators, but which are related to a larger construct.

A health status index might combine the values of many indicators into one measure. As a simple illustration, the low birthweight rates and the child injury mortality rates for the 10 counties will be combined. Here are the results for all 10 counties using integer ranks:

County	Integer Ranks for Low Birthweight Rate (%)		Integer Ranks for Child Injury Mortality Rate (per 100,000)		Index Scores of Health Status Mean of the 2 Ranks
A	1	(4.17)	7	(46.60)	4.0
B	2	(5.68)	6	(45.94)	4.0
C	3	(6.08)	8	(47.69)	5.5
D	4	(6.41)	3	(36.55)	3.5
E	5	(6.49)	10	(81.50)	7.5
F	6	(6.96)	2	(31.38)	4.0
G	7	(7.20)	5	(42.83)	6.0
H	8	(7.75)	4	(39.36)	6.0
I	9	(8.44)	1	(30.79)	5.0
J	10	(21.05)	9	(52.64)	9.5

Another index could be defined by combining a health status and a health services indicator to address a particular health problem. For example, the trend in a health status measure could be combined with the trend in the availability of relevant health services. Counties might then be assigned to one of the following categories:

1. health status improving, services constant or increasing
2. health status improving, services decreasing
3. health status deteriorating, services constant or increasing
4. health status deteriorating, services decreasing

In this index, the trend in health status is given precedence over the trend in available services; improvement or deterioration in the rate of occurrence is considered primary since health services are only one factor influencing any change in health status.

3. An index may combine variables which cross constructs, but which are related as dimensions of a larger, complex system.

A global index of MCH need might include measures of risk and of outcome, and also measures of access, availability and utilization of health services. In this scenario, a constellation of indicators is selected, index scores are generated to summarize all of the data, and geographic areas are grouped according to the index scores.

Selecting which component measures are to be used in constructing an index, and exactly how these measures will be used should be driven by a conceptual understanding of the relationship among indicators with respect to the particular issue being addressed. A given variable might be handled in any of several ways. For example, it might be:

- Used as one of the primary measures included in an index
- Used to standardize (adjust) the primary measures in an index
- Used to define strata of the component measures in an index
- Used to weight the component measures in an index
- Not used at all

Categorization, integer ranking, percentile rescaled values, z-scores, and z-tests may all be used in constructing indices. Once the selected measures have been transformed to a comparable scale, whether through creation of discrete or continuous scores, then an approach for combining the measures into a summary index can be developed.

As the examples above illustrated, the index itself may be categorical or continuous. If the component measures are categorized, then an algorithm can be developed to combine the categories into new ones. If the component measures are continuous scores, then an algorithm can be developed to combine these either into discrete categories or into a new set of continuous scores.

The algorithm is a set of rules for how to combine the component measures. Each component measure may be treated equally (unweighted) or differentially (weighted). If measures are to be weighted, usually the differential weights are defined conceptually, by considering the relative importance of each component measure in terms of, for example, the consequences of the outcome, how common it is, whether intervention strategies exist to address it, how effective the existing strategies are, and how feasible it is to implement interventions in terms of cost and other factors. If statistical procedures are used to combine measures, weighting may be part of the algorithm itself.

A typical algorithm for constructing an index is simply to sum (or compute the mean) of the scores across all of the component measures. If weighting is to be used, this is done either explicitly by multiplying each measure by its assigned weight prior to summing, or implicitly by defining discrete categories that result in summing across non-equivalent levels of each measure. Let's look at an example to see how this process works.

Suppose the index combining number of low birthweight births and the low birthweight rate seen earlier is created, but this time giving more weight to the low birthweight rate than to the number of low birthweight births. An explicit weight of 2 might be assigned to the rate, while the number of low birthweight births will have a weight of 1.

County	Integer Ranks for Number of Low Birthweight Births Weight=1		Integer Ranks for Low Birthweight Rate (%) Weight=2		Index Scores of Low Birthweight Mean of the 2 Ranks Weighted
A	2	(14)	2×1=2	(4.17)	2.0
B	10	(193)	2×2=4	(5.68)	7.0
C	5	(41)	2×3=6	(6.08)	5.5
D	9	(129)	2×4=8	(6.41)	8.5
E	1	(12)	2×5=10	(6.49)	5.5
F	4	(38)	2×6=12	(6.96)	8.0
G	8	(124)	2×7=14	(7.20)	11.0
H	7	(93)	2×8=16	(7.75)	11.5
I	6	(60)	2×9=18	(8.44)	12.0
J	3	(24)	2×10=20	(21.05)	11.5

The index scores are now somewhat different than before (refer to the table on page 163). County I now has the highest score, though not by very much. Counties G and H, which were tied before are now differentiated since County H's low birthweight rate is higher than County G's and this indicator is weighted more. In addition, these two counties are no longer scored higher than County J as they were when no weighting was applied. Finally, County D's score is relatively lower in comparison to the counties with the highest scores, because its large number of low birthweight births now has a diminished impact on the index score.

Now let's look at using discrete categories to implicitly weight the two indicators. The low birthweight rate will be divided into 5 categories with two counties in each (quintiles) and the number of low birthweight births into only 2 categories with five counties in each (below and above the median). Here are the results:

County	Median Ranks for Number of Low Birthweight Births		Quintile Ranks for Low Birthweight Rate (%)		Index Scores of Low Birthweight Mean of the 2 Ranks Weighted
A	1	(14)	1	(4.17)	1.0
B	2	(193)	1	(5.68)	1.5
C	1	(41)	2	(6.08)	1.5
D	2	(129)	2	(6.41)	2.0
E	1	(12)	3	(6.49)	2.0
F	1	(38)	3	(6.96)	2.0
G	2	(124)	4	(7.20)	3.0
H	2	(93)	4	(7.75)	3.0
I	2	(60)	5	(8.44)	3.5
J	1	(24)	5	(21.05)	3.0

Because the low birthweight rates are divided into more categories than the number of low birthweight births, they dominate the order of the index scores. The number of low birthweight births, however, has influenced the index scores somewhat. For instance, County D is tied with Counties E and F because, even though its low birthweight rate is lower, it is in the higher category for number of low birthweight births.

One final note on constructing indices: be careful before combining measures (or even before comparing measures), that the directionality of the indicators is comparable—make sure a high score on one measure has the equivalent meaning as a high score on another measure. On some indicators, such as number of physicians per capita in a community, a high score is "good" and a low score is "bad". Categories, ranks, rescaled values, and scores must reflect this. For example, the order of ranks for the number of physicians per capita and the signs (positive or negative) of z-scores or z-tests would have to be reversed in order to achieve consistency with other indicators such as low birthweight or child injury mortality. If this seeming detail is forgotten, index scores will be inaccurate and misleading.

You can see that there are a myriad of approaches to constructing indices. The analyst has a great deal of flexibility in accomplishing this task, but the underlying conceptual framework should not be allowed to get lost in the mechanical process.

Comment

Often, when summarizing data, multiple methods are used in combination. For example, several indicators with values for many geographic areas might first be rescaled to a common range, then combined into an index by calculating the mean of the rescaled values for each area, and finally turned into a few discrete categories with labels such as "areas in most need", "areas with moderate need", and "areas with least need".

Similarly, after initial ranking or scoring, an index might be constructed and then ranking or scoring might be applied again to the index values themselves.

Sometimes, two scoring methods are used at once to capture multiple perspectives: for instance, z-tests might be used to identify statistically significant departures from a standard, while integer ranks might be used as well to provide a more readily understood measure of relative position.

Mapping is often chosen as a presentation format to gain the advantages of index construction without losing the information on each component measure. The layering of information on the map in effect combines it into one composite measure, but the layers can be pealed away or re-combined (the index deconstructed or reconstructed) to yield slightly different views of the health issue being examined.

Index construction might also occur in stages. For example, indicators within given domains might be rescaled and combined into distinct indices, and then these indices may be combined into one grand summary measure. For example, one index might be created to summarize health status measures, one to summarize health services measures, and one to summarize sociodemographic measures. These indices could be reported separately or together.

SUMMARIZING DATA TO ALLOCATE RESOURCES

The results of data summarization are sometimes used as input into a formula for distribution of resources. Developing a distribution formula requires its own series of choices that correspond to conceptual, analytic, practical, and political considerations. Perhaps the most fundamental issue to be addressed is whether resources will be distributed according to the size of the population at risk, according to need as measured by "high" scores on indicators or indices, according to some combination of both population size and need, or according to a more complex method that accounts for other factors such as demographic characteristics, historical funding patterns, or status of the public health infrastructure.

For example, it might be decided to divide the resource pool into two portions such that funds are allocated separately, according to population size alone and according to population size weighted by need. The pool might be split evenly, or a 10-90 split, a 25-75 split, or some other division may be deemed appropriate. Unless population sizes across areas do not vary greatly, it is necessary to consider need on a per capita basis in order to insure equitable distribution of funds. It is possible, though, to leave the resource pool undivided, allocating 100% of the resources based on population size weighted by need.

It may also be important to designate a portion of the resource pool for funding areas that have a track record in implementing programs and policies that result in improved health status. These areas often score low on need indices and therefore are not targeted for infusion of resources. It can be argued, however, that their successes should be rewarded with funding, both to facilitate continued improvement, and as an incentive for other areas to adopt and adapt effective approaches.

In essence, developing a resource allocation formula is constructing an index, using whatever factors are considered relevant to the process. For example, all previously computed indicator or index scores might be rescaled to reflect the desired differential in weighting. Perhaps a range of 1 to 2 will be chosen so that the "worst" area receives twice the funding on a per capita basis as the "best" area. Perhaps a range of 1 to 5 will be chosen to increase the per capita differential in funding. Perhaps all areas will first be allocated a fixed amount based on population at risk and then only those areas whose z-scores are > 1 will be allocated additional funds based on excess need. Perhaps those areas with more than a 1% average annual increase (deterioration) and those with more than a 1% average annual decrease (improvement) will be given a weight of 2, while those areas with less than a 1% average annual change in either direction will be given a weight of only 1.

The resource allocation index or formula can also build-in rules that reflect political considerations. For instance, a baseline level of funding can be defined either in absolute dollars or relative to historical funding levels. The baseline might be defined so that no area receives less funding than it had in the past, or so that any decreases are limited to, say, a 5 or 10 % reduction. Similarly, a funding ceiling can be defined either in absolute dollars or relative to historical funding levels. The ceiling might be defined, for example, so that no area receives more than a 5 or 10% increase.

Suppose $2,000,000 is to be distributed to counties A through J for low birthweight prevention. In the past, this amount had been distributed based solely on the total number of births in each county. The following table shows the distribution of funds to each county according to its proportionate share of the 10,887 births that occurred in all ten counties combined:

County	Number of Births	% of Total Births	Funds Allocated ($)
A	336	3.1	62,000.00
B	3,397	31.2	624,000.00
C	674	6.2	124,000.00
D	2,013	18.5	370,000.00
E	185	1.7	34,000.00
F	546	5.0	100,000.00
G	1,723	15.8	316,000.00
H	1,200	11.0	220,000.00
I	699	6.4	128,000.00
J	114	1.0	20,000.00
TOTAL	10,887	100.0	~2,000,000.00

Now suppose that the following hypothetical rules for a new distribution formula are agreed upon:

1. Allocation of funds will be based on both population at risk and excess need as reflected in low birthweight z-tests.

2. All counties will receive funds from each category—the county with the smallest population will receive funds based on its population at risk and the county with the best low birthweight z-test will receive funds earmarked for excess need.

3. The $2,000,000.00 will be split evenly between population at risk and excess need, and the z-tests will be rescaled to a range of 1 to 2 so that no county will experience more than a 10 % reduction in resources.

The following table lays the basis for the distribution of funds according to the new rules:

County	a. Low Birthweight z-tests	b. # of Births	c. % of Total Births
A	-1.84	336	3.1
B	-2.33	3,397	31.2
C	-0.62	674	6.2
D	-0.48	2,013	18.5
E	-0.10	185	1.7
F	0.26	546	5.0
G	0.87	1,723	15.8
H	1.49	1,200	11.0
I	1.87	699	6.4
J	6.15	114	1.0
		10,887	100.0

(Table continued on next page)

County	d. Low Birthweight Rescaled z-tests	e. # of Births Weighted by Rescaled z-tests	f.* % of Total Births Weighted by Rescaled z-tests
A	1.06	356	2.7
B	1.00	3,397	25.4
C	1.20	809	6.1
D	1.22	2,456	18.4
E	1.25	231	1.7
F	1.31	715	5.4
G	1.38	2,378	17.8
H	1.45	1,740	13.0
I	1.50	1,049	7.9
J	2.00	228	1.7
		13,359	100.0

Column d. shows the z-tests rescaled to a range of 1 to 2 using the formula described on pages 150-151. County C's rescaled value of 1.20, for example, was calculated as follows:

County C

$$\frac{\text{New Value} - 1}{2 - 1} = \frac{-0.62 - (-2.33)}{6.15 - (-2.33)}$$

$$\text{New Value} - 1 = \frac{1.71}{8.48} \times 1$$

$$\text{New Value} = (0.20 \times 1) + 1$$

$$= 1.20$$

Column e. is the distribution of the populations at risk weighted by the rescaled z-tests. County C's weighted number of births, then, is calculated as $1.20 \times 674 = 809$ (column d. × column b.), and this is 6.1% of the weighted total ($(809 \div 13,359) \times 100$). Once these weighted percents are calculated for all 10 counties, the $2,000,000.000 can be allocated. Remember that half of the funds, or $1,000,000.00, will be allocated based solely on the population at risk and the other half will be allocated based on the z-tests weighted by the population at risk. The following table shows the results:

County	% of Total Births Unweighted	Funds Allocated Population at Risk ($)	% of Total Births Weighted by Rescaled z-tests	Funds Allocated Excess Need ($)
A	3.1	31,000.00	2.7	27,000.00
B	31.2	312,000.00	25.4	254,000.00
C	6.2	62,000.00	6.1	61,000.00
D	18.5	185,000.00	18.4	184,000.00
E	1.7	17,000.00	1.7	17,000.00
F	5.0	50,000.00	5.4	54,000.00
G	15.8	158,000.00	17.8	178,000.00
H	11.0	110,000.00	13.0	130,000.00
I	6.4	64,000.00	7.9	79,000.00
J	1.0	10,000.00	1.7	17,000.00
	100.0	~1,000,000.00	100.0	~1,000,000.00

After summing the funds allocated to each county from both halves of the resource pool, here is the comparison between the old and the new distribution:

County	Previous Allocation of Funds ($) Population at Risk Only	New Allocation of Funds ($) Population at Risk and Need 50-50 Split
A	62,000.00	58,000.00
B	624,000.00	566,000.00
C	124,000.00	123,000.00
D	370,000.00	369,000.00
E	34,000.00	34,000.00
F	100,000.00	104,000.00
G	316,000.00	336,000.00
H	220,000.00	240,000.00
I	128,000.00	143,000.00
J	20,000.00	27,000.00
	~2,000,000.00	~2,000,000.00

The hypothetical rules agreed upon for distributing funds were quite conservative, resulting in fairly minor differences from the old method. Counties A-C, with the lowest low birthweight rates would receive a slight decrease in funds, while Counties H-J, with the highest low birthweight rates would receive a slight increase in funds.

If a greater proportion of funds had been allocated based on excess need, if decreases and increases in funding had not been limited, and/or if the z-tests had been scaled to a range greater than 1-2, the results would have shown more pronounced differences compared to the old method. For example, if 100% of the funds were allocated based on the rescaled z-tests for the low birthweight rates, the results would be as follows:

County	Previous Allocation of Funds ($) Population at Risk Only	New Allocation of Funds ($) Population at Risk and Need 0-100 Split
A	62,000.00	54,000.00
B	624,000.00	508,000.00
C	124,000.00	122,000.00
D	370,000.00	368,000.00
E	34,000.00	34,000.00
F	100,000.00	104,000.00
G	316,000.00	356,000.00
H	220,000.00	260,000.00
I	128,000.00	158,000.00
J	20,000.00	34,000.00
	~2,000,000.00	~2,000,000.00

Now the shift in funding is greater, but the hypothetical rules have been violated. In order to increase funds to Counties H-J with their elevated low birthweight rates, the funding of Counties A and B is reduced by more than 10%—County A's funding is reduced by more than $6,200.00 and County B's funding is reduced by more than $62,400.00. Once again, analytic choices greatly influence results and must always be made with care and with a sound rationale that is developed through a broad based consensus building process.

SUMMARY

Summarizing data is a complex process, with summarization occurring within and across many dimensions simultaneously and sequentially. A well structured analysis plan is essential for controlling the process and insuring that the final product reflects the analytic goals. The data burden can be reduced both by limiting the amount of data used and by applying methods to increase the interpretability of the data. Categorizing, ranking, scoring, indexing, and multivariable statistical methods are tools for increasing the interpretability of data, as are graphing, mapping, and other presentation methods.

It is critical to state the assumptions and acknowledge the overall strategies that drive the choice of analytic methods and presentation formats. Different choices can lead to different results and potentially to different conclusions. It is essential, therefore, to examine the impact of, and the tradeoffs, that each choice carries with it. Sensitivity analysis—contrasting the results achieved using differing sets of choices—is strongly recommended.

Data summarization is not an end in itself. Its purpose is to achieve a coherent view of health problems—a view that, in maternal and child health, promotes action to improve the health of women, infants, children, adolescents, and families.

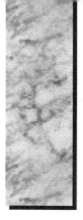

Methods for Summarizing Data Exercise and Solution

Suppose that you are the director of the Office of Planning and Evaluation for the state's Bureau of Maternal and Child Health. It is an election year and the legislature has just approved an additional $2,000,000.00 for improving maternal and child health in ten select counties in the state. Your office is asked to identify the counties in the most "need" and to design a resource allocation strategy.

The following pages contain data on several MCH indicators for the ten counties. A data dictionary describing each indicator is also provided.

In addition to the original indicator values, integer ranks, z-scores, and z-tests have been computed for the 10 counties. Some of these values, however, are missing and will have to be calculated in order to obtain a complete set of ranks/scores for a particular indicator. Indicator means and standard deviations as well as aggregate population numerators and denominators are provided.

The purpose of the exercise is to summarize some or all of the indicators provided as part of a hypothetical MCH/CSHCN planning and assessment process. The following instructions are not intended as hard and fast rules, but are merely intended as an aid in the decisionmaking process.

Instructions

1. Use all or some of the indicators. It is recommended that at least 5 should be used.
2. Create one or more summary measures, or justify why indicators will be addressed separately. Discuss the results.
3. Translate the indicators or summary measure(s) into a resource allocation formula. Discuss the results.

Things to Keep in Mind

1. Directionality of an indicator. What is the meaning of "high" or "low"? The ranks/scores have been computed with this in mind.
2. Should each indicator be given equal weight?
3. How should population size be incorporated?
4. The indicator labeled "Distance", unlike the other indicators, is a dichotomous variable (yes or no) and as such may have to be handled in a somewhat different fashion.

Data Dictionary

Label*	Variable	Definition / Data Source
COUNTY		
TOTPOP	# Total Population	Census
A17	# Children Under 18	Census
BTHS	# Births	Vital Records
SN17	# CSHCN Clients Served	CSHCN Program Data
DISTANCE	Distance to Specialty Care	Average Distance >50 Miles—Yes or No
LBWR	Low Birthweight Rate %	# Low Birthweight Births per 100 births
IDTHSR	Infant Mortality Rate	# Infant Deaths per 1000 Births
B10T17R	% Teen Births	# Births to Teens per 100 Births
NOPCR	% with No Prenatal Care	# Women with no PNC per 100 Births
EPSDTR	EPSDT Coverage Rate (%)	# Served by EPSDT per 100 Children in Poverty
PARENTS	% Satisfied with Care Coordination	# Satisfied per 100 CSHCN clients
PHYSR	Physician Rate	# Physicians per 1000 Total Population
PV17R	Child Poverty Rate (%)	# < 18 in Poverty per 100 Children <18
DELIVR	% Medicaid (XIX) Deliveries	# Deliveries Paid by XIX per 100 Births
INJURYR	Child Injury Mortality Rate	# Injuries per 100,000 Children < 18
CABUSER	Child Abuse/Neglect Rate	# Reported Cases per 1000 Children < 18

- The variable labels will be prefaced with "Z1" for the z-scores, and with "Z2" for the z-tests.

DESCRIPTIVE STATISTICS

Variable	Indicator for the 10 Counties Combined (Weighted Mean)	Mean of the 10 County Indicators (Unweighted Mean)	Standard Deviation of the County Indicators
LBWR	6.68	8.02	4.72
IDTHSR	9.92	10.83	3.77
B10T17R	5.70	5.37	1.48
NOPCR	1.10	1.17	0.26
EPSDTR	78.50	74.13	11.60
PARENTS	73.83	73.45	10.53
PHYSR	1.58	1.32	0.60
PV17R	18.50	19.90	8.31
DELIVR	38.97	36.62	8.54
INJURYR	42.77	45.52	14.50
CABUSER	53.48	45.75	15.67

Summarizing Data
Select MCH/CSHCN Indicators

COUNTY	TOTPOP TOTAL POPULATION	A17 CHILD POPULATION	PV17 CHILDREN IN POVERTY	BTHS BIRTHS	SN17 CSHCN CLIENTS	DISTANCE TO SPECIALTY CARE > 50 MILES
1	14991	3681	506	185	69	1
2	31704	9559	1105	546	154	1
3	30787	7971	932	336	85	0
4	61067	11600	3090	699	254	0
5	56393	13480	2590	674	157	0
6	117206	30407	5768	1723	507	0
7	249238	63748	10454	3397	941	1
8	7523	2171	856	114	96	0
9	148723	37909	7223	2013	354	0
10	88257	22868	5104	1200	390	
	805889	203394	37628	10887	3007	

COUNTY	LBWR	IDTHSR	B10T17R	NOPCR	EPSDTR	PARENTS	PHYSR	PV17R	DELIVR	INJURYR	CABUSER
1	6.49	16.22	3.78	1.08	84.58	89.2	0.73	13.75	36.76	81.50	42.65
2	6.96	12.82	2.75	1.10	71.76	69.0	1.51	11.56	21.98	31.38	33.27
3	4.17	8.93	6.55	0.89	69.53	66.0	0.71	11.69	22.62	46.60	16.81
4	8.44	11.44	4.15	1.14	65.24	52.0	1.98	26.64	37.20	30.79	42.07
5	6.08	10.39	5.79	1.48	80.77	83.6	1.51	19.21	35.31	47.69	49.93
6	7.20	7.54	7.02	1.10	85.26	73.5	1.80	18.97	42.54	42.83	57.75
7	5.68	6.77	4.77	1.03	87.38	76.2	1.48	16.40	39.51	45.94	51.64
8	21.05	17.54	5.26	1.75	48.71	71.0	0.13	39.43	42.98	52.64	31.78
9	6.41	9.94	6.86	1.19	72.28	71.0	1.86	19.05	38.10	36.55	65.26
10	7.75	6.67	6.75	0.92	75.84	83.0	1.45	22.32	49.17	39.36	66.29

Summarizing Data
Integer Ranks

COUNTY	TOTPOP TOTAL POPULATION	A17 CHILD POPULATION	PV17 CHILDREN IN POVERTY	BTHS BIRTHS	SN17 CSHCN CLIENTS	DISTANCE TO SPECIALTY CARE > 50 MILES
1	14991	3681	506	185	69	1
2	31704	9559	1105	546	154	1
3	30787	7971	932	336	85	0
4	61067	11600	3090	699	254	0
5	56393	13480	2590	674	157	0
6	117206	30407	5768	1723	507	0
7	249238	63748	10454	3397	941	0
8	7523	2171	856	114	96	1
9	148723	37909	7223	2013	354	0
10	88257	22868	5104	1200	390	0
	805889	203394	37628	10887	3007	

COUNTY	LBWR	IDTHSR	B10T17R	NOPCR	EPSDTR	PARENTS	PHYSR	PV17R	DELIVR	INJURYR	CABUSER
1	5	9	2	4	3	1	8	3	4	10	5
2	6		1	5.5		8	4.5	1	1	2	
3	1	4		1	8	9	9		2	7	1
4	9	7	3	7	9	10	1	9	5	1	4
5	3	6	6	9	4	2	4.5	7	3	8	6
6	7		10	5.5		5	3	5	8	5	
7	2	2	4	3	1	4	6	4	7	6	7
8	10	10	5	10	10	6.5	10	10	9	9	2
9	4	5		8	6	6.5			6	3	9
10	8	1	8	2	5	3	7	8	10	4	10

Summarizing Data
Z-Scores

COUNTY	TOTPOP TOTAL POPULATION	A17 CHILD POPULATION	PV17 CHILDREN IN POVERTY	BTHS BIRTHS	SN17 CSHCN CLIENTS	DISTANCE TO SPECIALTY CARE > 50 MILES
1	14991	3681	506	185	69	1
2	31704	9559	1105	546	154	1
3	30787	7971	932	336	85	0
4	61067	11600	3090	699	254	0
5	56393	13480	2590	674	157	0
6	117206	30407	5768	1723	507	0
7	249238	63748	10454	3397	941	0
8	7523	2171	856	114	96	1
9	148723	37909	7223	2013	354	0
10	88257	22868	5104	1200	390	0
	======	======	=====	=====	====	
	805889	203394	37628	10887	3007	

COUNTY	Z1LBW	Z1DTH	Z1TEEN	Z1PNC	Z1SDT	Z1PAR	Z1DOC	Z1POV	Z1DEL
1	-0.32	1.43	-1.07	-0.34	-0.90	-1.50	0.98	-0.74	0.02
2	-0.23		-1.77	-0.26		0.42	-0.32	-1.00	-1.71
3	-0.82	-0.50		-1.07	0.40	0.71	-1.11	0.81	-1.64
4	0.09	0.16	-0.82	-0.11	0.77	2.04	-0.32	-0.08	0.07
5	-0.41	-0.12	0.29	1.20	-0.57	-0.96	-0.81	-0.11	-0.15
6	-0.17		1.12	-0.26		0.00	-0.27	-0.42	0.69
7	-0.50	-1.08	-0.40	-0.53	-1.14	-0.26			0.34
8	2.76	1.78	-0.07	2.23	2.19	0.23	1.99	2.35	0.75
9	-0.34	-0.24		0.08	0.16	0.23			0.17
10	-0.06	-1.10	0.94	-0.95	-0.15	-0.91	-0.22	0.29	1.47

Summarizing Data
Z-Tests

COUNTY	TOTPOP TOTAL POPULATION	A17 CHILD POPULATION	PV17 CHILDREN IN POVERTY	BTHS BIRTHS	SN17 CSHCN CLIENTS	DISTANCE TO SPECIALTY CARE > 50 MILES
1	14991	3681	506	185	69	1
2	31704	9559	1105	546	154	1
3	30787	7971	932	336	85	0
4	61067	11600	3090	699	254	0
5	56393	13480	2590	674	157	0
6	117206	30407	5768	1723	507	0
7	249238	63748	10454	3397	941	0
8	7523	2171	856	114	96	1
9	148723	37909	7223	2013	354	0
10	88257	22868	5104	1200	390	0
	======	======	=====	=====	====	
	805889	203394	37628	10887	3007	

COUNTY	Z2LBW	Z2DTH	Z2TEEN	Z2PNC	Z2SDT	Z2PAR	Z2DOC	Z2POV	Z2DEL
1	-0.10	0.86	-1.12	-0.03	-3.33	-2.90	2.62	-7.44	-0.62
2	0.26		-2.97	0.00		1.36	0.31	-17.52	-8.14
3	-1.84	-0.18	-1.76	-0.37	6.67	1.64			-6.14
4	1.87	0.40	0.11	0.10	17.94	7.91	-2.49	22.64	-0.96
5	-0.62	0.12		0.94	-2.81	-2.78	0.42	2.13	-1.95
6	0.87		2.37	-0.01		0.17	-1.89	2.12	3.03
7	-2.33	-1.84	-2.33	-0.40	-22.10	-1.65	1.26	-13.69	0.64
8	6.15	0.82	-0.20	0.66	21.21	0.63	3.16	25.18	0.88
9	-0.48	0.01		0.38	12.87	1.21			-0.80
10	1.49	-1.13	1.58	-0.60	4.63	-4.12	0.97	14.92	7.24

Two Possible Solutions for
Summarizing Data Exercise

Looking at the many values provided for the 10 counties, it is extremely difficult to discern an overall pattern of need, assess overall relative standing, or devise a rational funding strategy. In the solutions presented here, indicators will first be summarized into 3 indices of need; the first index will summarize health status indicators, the second will summarize indicators related to health services, and the third will summarize demographic indicators. All but one of the indicators provided will be used in one of these 3 indices. The indicator for child abuse/neglect will not be used because of potential reporting problems within and across counties that might compromise its accuracy.

1. Health Status Index
   Low Birthweight Rate (%)
   Infant Mortality Rate (per 1,000)
   % Teen Births
   Child Injury Mortality

2. Health Services Index
   No Prenatal Care (%)
   EPSDT Coverage Rate (%)
   CSHCN Parent Satisfaction (%)
   Physicians per 1,000 Total Population
   Distance to Specialty Care (> 50 miles, yes or no)

3, Demographic Index
   Child Poverty Rate (%)
   % Deliveries Paid by Medicaid

Both the integer ranks and z-test results provided for the indicators will be used. A county's score on each index will be the mean of these ranks or z-test results for the component measures. Counties identified as in the most need according to each index will be reported. The raw index scores will then be rescaled to a range of 0-2 and will be used in this form to weight the child population of each county in the construction of a resource distribution formula.

Solution 1:

The $2,000,000 will be divided into 4 segments: $500,000 will be allocated according to the actual distribution of the child population across the 10 counties, $500,000 will be allocated according to the distribution of the child population weighted by the health status index, $500,000 will be allocated according to the distribution of the child population weighted by the health services index, and $500,000 will be allocated according to the distribution of the child population weighted by the demographic index.

Solution 2:

The $2,000,000 will be divided into 2 segments: $1,000,000 will be allocated according to the actual distribution of the child population across the 10 counties, and $1,000,000 will be allocated according to the distribution of the child population weighted by the health status index. The other two indices will not be incorporated into the funding formula.

Each solution is presented twice: using integer ranks and z-tests.

These solutions are offered as suggestions. There are countless other ways that the data could be organized and a funding formula developed. For example, instead of combining indicators of the same type (e.g., health status indicators), indices might be organized around target populations yielding an Infant Health Index, a Child Health Index, or a Children with Special Health Care Needs Index. Even with the indices created here, the assignment of certain indicators might be changed; for instance, % teen births could be included in the Demographic Index rather than the Health Status Index, or % no prenatal care could be included in the Health Status Index rather than in the Health Services Index. In addition, total population, child population in poverty, or number of live births could be used rather than the total child population as the foundation for the funding formula.

Using the 3 indices and the two approaches to allocating resources described above, here are the necessary calculations and results. Tables 1a., 1b., and 1c. show the scores on the three need indices, based on integer ranks and also on z-test results:

| County | Table 1a. Health Status Index Score | |
	Integer Ranks	z-tests
1	6.50	0.66
2	4.25	-0.87
3	4.75	-0.23
4	5.00	-0.29
5	5.75	0.09
6	6.25	0.57
7	3.50	-1.37
8	8.50	1.84
9	5.25	0.06
10	5.25	0.32

Example: For County 1, the Health Status Index score is calculated as follows:

Integer Ranks

z - tests

$$\frac{5+9+2+10}{4} = 6.5 \quad \text{or} \quad \frac{-0.10 + 0.86 + (-1.12) + 3.01}{4} = 0.66$$

| County | Table 1b. Health Services Index Score | |
	Integer Ranks	z-tests
1	4.25	-0.66
2	6.50	2.03
3	6.75	2.95
4	6.75	5.87
5	4.88	-1.06
6	3.88	-3.56
7	3.50	-5.72
8	9.38	6.67
9	5.63	2.94
10	4.25	0.22

Example: For County 1, the Health Services Index score is calculated as follows:

Integer Ranks   z - tests

$$\frac{4+3+1+8+1}{4}=4.25 \quad \text{or} \quad \frac{-0.03+(-3.33)+(-2.90)+2.62+1}{4}=-0.66$$

Notice that although there are 5 component measures included in this index, the mean is calculated using a denominator of 4. This is simply a way of differentiating the indicator labeled "Distance" from the others. A "1" on this indicator does not have the same meaning as either an integer rank of 1 or a z-test result of 1.

County	Table 1c. Demographic Index Score	
	Integer Ranks	z-tests
1	3.50	-4.03
2	1.00	-12.83
3	2.00	-10.92
4	7.00	10.84
5	5.00	0.09
6	6.50	2.58
7	5.50	-6.52
8	9.50	13.03
9	6.00	0.98
10	9.00	11.08

Example: For County 1, the Demographic Index score is calculated as follows:

Integer Ranks   z - tests

$$\frac{3+4}{2}=3.5 \quad \text{or} \quad \frac{-7.44+(-0.62)}{2}=-4.03$$

Tables 2 and 3 (using integer ranks and z-tests respectively) show the counties sorted according to the size of their child population and their scores on the three need indices.

Table 2

Counties Ordered from the Largest to the Smallest Child population	Counties Ordered from the Highest to the Lowest Index Scores Based on Integer Ranks (Most Need to Least Need)		
	Health Status	Health Services	Demographic
County 7	County 8	County 8	County 8
9	1	4 and 3	10
6	6		4
10	5	2	6
5	10 and 9	9	9
4		5	7
2	4	10 and 1	5
3	3		1
1	2	6	3
8	7	7	2

Table 3

Counties Ordered from the Largest to the Smallest Child population	Counties Ordered from the Highest to the Lowest Index Scores Based on z-tests (Most Need to Least Need)		
	Health Status	Health Services	Demographic
County 7	County 8	County 8	County 8
9	1	4	10
6	6	3	4
10	10	9	6
5	5	2	9
4	9	10	5
2	3	1	1
3	4	5	7
1	2	6	3
8	7	7	2

Summarized into the indices, it is now easier to identify County 8 as performing poorly on many health measures in comparison to the other 9 counties, although it has the smallest child population. County 7, on the other hand, has the largest child population, and is performing well on the indicators provided. Counties 8, 1, and 6 have the greatest need according to the Health Status Index, counties 8, 4, and 3 have the greatest need according to the Health Services Index, and counties 8, 10, and 4 have the greatest need according to the Demographic Index. Counties 4, 6, 9, and 10 are among the counties with the greatest need and also have substantial child population size.

Also, notice that the sorted order on the indices is somewhat different depending on whether integer ranks or z-tests are used. With z-tests, it is also possible to divide the counties according to those with average z-test results above (worse) or below (better) the overall indicator value for the ten counties combined. Using this information, County 9, although not one of the three counties in greatest need according to the indices, has average z-test results greater than 0 (worse than the overall indicators) on all three indices, and in addition has the second largest child population of the ten counties, Tables 4a., 4b., and 4c. show the scores on the three need indices rescaled to a range of 0-2, based on integer ranks and also on z-test results:

| County | Table 4a. Health Status Index Score | |
| | Integer Ranks | z-tests |
	Rescaled To A Range Of 0-2	
1	1.2	1.26
2	0.3	0.31
3	0.5	0.71
4	0.6	0.67
5	0.9	0.91
6	1.1	1.21
7	0.0	0.00
8	2.0	2.00
9	0.7	0.89
10	0.7	1.05

Example: For County 1, the rescaled Health Status Index score is calculated as follows:

Integer Ranks

$$\frac{\text{New Value} - 0}{2 - 0} = \frac{6.5 - 3.5}{8.5 - 3.5}$$

or

z - tests

$$\frac{\text{New Value} - 0}{2 - 0} = \frac{0.66 - (-1.37)}{1.84 - (-1.37)}$$

$$\text{New Value} - 0 = \frac{3}{5} \times (2 - 0)$$

$$\text{New Value} - 0 = \frac{2.03}{3.21} \times (2 - 0)$$

$$\text{New Value} = 1.2$$

$$\text{New Value} = 1.26$$

| County | Table 4b. Health Services Index Score | |
| | Integer Ranks | z-tests |
	Rescaled To A Range Of 0-2	
1	0.26	0.82
2	1.02	1.25
3	1.11	1.40
4	1.11	1.87
5	0.47	0.75
6	0.13	0.35
7	0.00	0.00
8	2.00	2.00
9	0.72	1.40
10	0.26	0.96

Example: For County 1, the rescaled Health Services Index score is calculated as follows:

Integer Ranks

z - tests

$$\frac{\text{New Value} - 0}{2 - 0} = \frac{4.25 - 3.5}{9.38 - 3.5} \quad \text{or} \quad \frac{\text{New Value} - 0}{2 - 0} = \frac{-0.66 - (-5.72)}{6.67 - (-5.72)}$$

$$\text{New Value} - 0 = \frac{0.75}{5.88} \times (2 - 0) \qquad \text{New Value} - 0 = \frac{5.06}{12.39} \times (2 - 0)$$

$$\text{New Value} = 0.26 \qquad\qquad \text{New Value} = 0.82$$

County	Table 4c. Demographic Index Score	
	Integer Ranks	z-tests
	Rescaled To A Range Of 0-2	
1	0.59	0.68
2	0.00	0.00
3	0.24	0.15
4	1.41	1.83
5	0.94	1.00
6	1.29	1.19
7	1.06	0.49
8	2.00	2.00
9	1.18	1.07
10	1.88	1.85

Example: For County 1, the rescaled Demographic Index score is calculated as follows:

Integer Ranks

z - tests

$$\frac{\text{New Value} - 0}{2 - 0} = \frac{3.5 - 1.0}{9.5 - 1.0} \quad \text{or} \quad \frac{\text{New Value} - 0}{2 - 0} = \frac{-4.03 - (-12.83)}{13.03 - (-12.83)}$$

$$\text{New Value} - 0 = \frac{2.5}{8.5} \times (2 - 0) \qquad \text{New Value} - 0 = \frac{8.8}{25.86} \times (2 - 0)$$

$$\text{New Value} = 0.59 \qquad\qquad \text{New Value} = 0.68$$

Next, Tables 5a., 5b., and 5c. show the distribution of the child (< 18) population across the 10 counties, unweighted (actual) and then weighted by the 0-2 scaled index scores.

Table 5a.						
Distribution of the Child Population						
COUNTY	Unweighted		Weighted by Health Status Index Scores			
			Rescaled Integer Ranks		Rescaled z-tests	
	n	%	n	%	n	%
1	3,681	1.8	4,417	4.0	4,638	3.5
2	9,559	4.7	2,868	2.6	2,963	2.2
3	7,971	3.9	3,986	3.6	5,659	4.3
4	11,600	5.7	6,960	6.3	7,772	5.9
5	13,480	6.6	12,132	11.0	12,267	9.3
6	30,407	14.9	33,448	30.2	36,792	27.8
7	63,748	31.3	0	0.0	0	0.0
8	2,171	1.1	4,342	3.9	4,342	3.3
9	37,909	18.6	26,536	24.0	33,739	25.5
10	22,868	11.2	16,008	14.5	24,011	18.2
TOTAL	203,394	100.0	110,697	100.0	132,183	100.0

Table 5b.						
Distribution of the Child Population						
COUNTY	Unweighted		Weighted by Health Services Index Scores			
			Rescaled Integer Ranks		Rescaled z-tests	
	n	%	n	%	n	%
1	3,681	1.8	957	1.2	3,018	2.0
2	9,559	4.7	9,750	12.1	11,949	8.1
3	7,971	3.9	8,848	11.0	11,159	7.5
4	11,600	5.7	12,876	16.0	21,692	14.7
5	13,480	6.6	6,336	7.9	10,110	6.8
6	30,407	14.9	3,953	4.9	10,642	7.2
7	63,748	31.3	0	0.0	0	0.0
8	2,171	1.1	4,342	5.4	4,342	2.9
9	37,909	18.6	27,294	34.0	53,073	35.9
10	22,868	11.2	5,946	7.4	21,953	14.8
TOTAL	203,394	100.0	80,302	100.0	147,938	100.0

Table 5c.						
Distribution of Child Population						
COUNTY	Unweighted		Weighted by Demographic Index Scores			
			Rescaled Integer Ranks		Rescaled z-tests	
	n	%	n	%	n	%
1	3,681	1.8	2,172	0.9	2,503	1.3
2	9,559	4.7	0	0.0	0	0.0
3	7,971	3.9	1,913	0.8	1,196	0.6
4	11,600	5.7	16,356	7.1	21,228	11.0
5	13,480	6.6	12,671	5.5	13,480	7.0
6	30,407	14.9	39,225	16.9	36,184	18.7
7	63,748	31.3	67,573	29.1	31,237	16.2
8	2,171	1.1	4,342	1.9	4,342	2.2
9	37,909	18.6	44,733	19.3	40,563	21.0
10	22,868	11.2	42,992	18.5	42,306	21.9
TOTAL	203,394	100.0	231,977	100.0	193,039	100.0

The weighted child population is determined by multiplying the rescaled index score for each county by the actual (unweighted) child population of each county. For County 1, using integer ranks, the weighted child population in County 1 is calculated as follows:

Health Status	$1.2 \times 3,681 = 4,417$, and $4,417 \div 110,697 = 0.040$ or 4.0%
Health Services	$0.26 \times 3,681 = 957$, and $957 \div 80,302 = 0.012$ or 1.2%
Demographic	$0.59 \times 3,681 = 2,172$, and $2,172 \div 231,977 = 0.009$ or 0.9%

Having adjusted the distribution of the child population to reflect relative need, the funds can be distributed accordingly. The first solution for allocating dollars is shown in tables 6a. and 6b., based on integer ranks and z-test results respectively.

Table 6a. Dollars Distributed To Each County Solution #1: Population And All 3 Indices Integer Ranks					
County	Unweighted	Weighted Status	Weighted Services	Weighted Demographic	TOTAL
1	$ 9,000.00	$ 20,000.00	$ 6,000.00	$ 4,500.00	$ 39,500.00
2	23,500.00	13,000.00	60,500.00	0.00	97,500.00
3	19,500.00	18,000.00	55,000.00	4,000.00	96,500.00
4	28,500.00	31,500.00	80,000.00	35,500.00	175,500.00
5	33,000.00	55,000.00	39,500.00	27,500.00	155,000.00
6	74,500.00	151,000.00	24,500.00	84,500.00	334,500.00
7	156,500.00	0.00	0.00	145,500.00	302,000.00
8	5,500.00	19,500.00	27,000.00	9,500.00	61,500.00
9	93,000.00	120,000.00	170,000.00	96,500.00	479,500.00
10	56,000.00	72,500.00	37,000.00	92,500.00	258,000.00
TOTAL	~$500,000.00	~$500,000.00	~$500,000.00	~$500,000.00	~$2,000,000.00

Table 6b. Dollars Distributed To Each County Solution #1: Population And All 3 Indices z-tests					
County	Unweighted	Wwighted Status	Weighted Services	Weighted Demographic	Total
1	$ 9,000.00	$ 17,500.00	$ 10,000.00	$ 6,500.00	$ 43,000.00
2	23,500.00	11,000.00	40,500.00	0.00	75,000.00
3	19,500.00	21,500.00	37,500.00	3,000.00	80,500.00
4	28,500.00	29,500.00	73,500.00	55,000.00	186,500.00
5	33,000.00	46,500.00	34,000.00	35,000.00	148,500.00
6	74,500.00	139,000.00	36,000.00	93,500.00	343,000.00
7	156,500.00	0.00	0.00	81,000.00	237,500.00
8	5,500.00	16,500.00	14,500.00	11,000.00	47,500.00
9	93,000.00	127,500.00	179,500.00	105,000.00	505,500.00
10	56,000.00	91,000.00	74,000.00	109,500.00	330,500.00
TOTAL	~$500,000.00	~$500,000.00	~$500,000.00	~$500,000.00	~$2,000,000.00

The dollars that will be allocated to each county using the child population and all 3 indices are determined by multiplying the unweighted or weighted percent by the appropriate pool of resources. For County 1, using integer ranks, the total amount of dollars is calculated as follows:

Population	$0.018 \times \$500,000 = \$\ 9,000.00$
Status	$0.04\ \ \times \$500,000 = \$20,000.00$
Services	$0.012 \times \$500,000 = \$\ 6,000.00$
Demographic	$0.009 \times \$500,000 = \$\ 4,500.00$
	========
Total	$\$39,500.00$

The second solution for allocating dollars is shown in tables 7a. and 7b., based on integer ranks and z-test results respectively.

Table 7a. Dollars Distributed To Each County Solution #2: Population And All 3 Indices Integer Ranks			
County	Unweighted	Weighted Status	TOTAL
1	$ 18,000.00	$ 40,000.00	$ 58,000.00
2	47,000.00	26,000.00	73,000.00
3	39,000.00	36,000.00	75,000.00
4	57,000.00	63,000.00	120,000.00
5	66,000.00	110,000.00	176,000.00
6	149,000.00	302,000.00	451,000.00
7	313,000.00	0.00	313,000.00
8	11,000.00	39,000.00	50,000.00
9	186,000.00	240,000.00	426,000.00
10	112,000.00	145,000.00	257,000.00
TOTAL	~$1,000,000.00	~$1,000,000.00	~$2,000,000.00

Table 7b. Dollars Distributed To Each County Solution #2: Population And All 3 Indices z-tests			
County	Unweighted	Wwighted Status	Total
1	$ 18,000.00	$ 35,000.00	$ 53,000.00
2	47,000.00	22,000.00	69,000.00
3	39,000.00	43,000.00	82,000.00
4	57,000.00	59,000.00	116,000.00
5	66,000.00	93,000.00	159,000.00
6	149,000.00	278,000.00	427,000.00
7	313,000.00	0.00	313,000.00
8	11,000.00	33,000.00	44,000.00
9	186,000.00	255,000.00	441,000.00
10	112,000.00	182,000.00	294,000.00
TOTAL	~$1,000,000.00	~$1,000,000.00	~$2,000,000.00

Following is a summary of how funds would be distributed according to Solution #1 and Solution #2, using either integer ranks or z-test results. Table 8a. shows the dollar amounts, and Table 8b. shows the percent distribution of the dollar amounts compared to the percent distribution of the actual child population across the 10 counties.

Table 8a.

County	Solution #1 Distribution of Dollars Population & Need All 3 Indices		Solution #2 Distribution of Dollars Population & Need Health Status Index Only	
	Integer Ranks	z-tests	Integer Ranks	z-tests
1	$ 39,500.00	$ 43,000.00	$ 58,000.00	$ 53,000.00
2	97,500.00	75,000.00	73,000.00	69,000.00
3	96,500.00	80,500.00	75,000.00	82,000.00
4	175,500.00	186,500.00	120,000.00	116,000.00
5	155,000.00	148,500.00	176,000.00	159,000.00
6	334,500.00	343,000.00	451,000.00	427,000.00
7	302,000.00	237,500.00	313,000.00	313,000.00
8	61,500.00	47,500.00	50,000.00	44,000.00
9	479,500.00	505,500.00	426,000.00	441,000.00
10	258,000.00	330,500.00	257,000.00	294,000.00
TOTAL	~$2,000,000.00	~$2,000,000.00	~$2,000,000.00	~$2,000,000.00

Table 8b.

County	% Distribution of Child Population	Solution #1 % Distribution of Dollars Population & Need All 3 Indices		Solution #2 % Distribution of Dollars Population & Need Health Status Index Only	
		Integer Ranks	z-tests	Integer Ranks	z-tests
1	1.8	2.0	2.2	2.9	2.7
2	4.7	4.9	3.8	3.7	3.5
3	3.9	4.8	4.0	3.8	4.1
4	5.7	8.8	9.3	6.0	5.8
5	6.6	7.8	7.4	8.8	8.0
6	14.9	16.7	17.2	22.6	21.4
7	31.3	15.1	11.9	15.7	15.7
8	1.1	3.1	2.4	2.5	2.2
9	18.6	24.0	25.3	21.3	22.1
10	11.2	12.9	16.5	12.9	14.7
TOTAL	~100.0	~100.0	~100.0	~100.0	~100.0

The way in which the $2,000,000 is segmented, the use of different indices, and the use of integer ranks or z-test results all have an impact on the final distribution of funds across the 10 counties. Although different methods yield different results, the general pattern is the same: County 7, which performed best on all three indices is given less funding relative to the size of its population, County 8, which performed the worst, is given more relative funding. Other counties also receive adjusted proportions of funding. Assuming that stakeholders have been involved in the process of developing the funding strategy, the results will be considered "fair" and can be implemented.

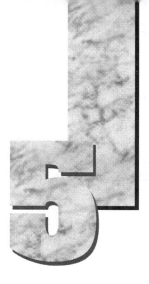

Methods for Analyzing Trend Data

by Deborah Rosenberg, PhD

A version of this module is available under the title "Trend Analysis And Interpretation: Key Concepts And Methods For Maternal And Child Health Professionals", a manuscript developed under a subcontract with the Public Health Foundation, Maternal and Child Health Information Resource Center, No. 240-94-0047. Funded by the Maternal and Child Health Bureau.

Public health agencies have a long tradition of monitoring trends in rates of disease and death and trends in medical, social, and behavioral risk factors that may contribute to these adverse events. Trends in observed rates provide invaluable information for needs assessment, program planning, program evaluation, and policy development activities. Examining data over time also permits making predictions about future frequencies and rates of occurrence.

Typically in public health, trend data are presented for rates arising from large populations over relatively long periods of time (e.g., ten or more years). For example, the national vital records system is a source for trend analysis of infant mortality and other death rates. The national rates described in these analyses are very reliable and are available over many years insuring a precise characterization of changes over time. These rates are considered as the true underlying population parameters and therefore statistical assessment, which implies that the data are subject to sampling error, is rarely undertaken. If rates are assumed to be error-free, they can be presented "as is" in tables or graphs, and comparisons across populations or predictions of future occurrence can be made intuitively.

In contrast to descriptive trend analysis, research studies of changes over time have followed a somewhat different analytic course. Because research data are usually sample data, statistical procedures, including sophisticated approaches such as time series analysis and formal forecasting techniques, are commonly used. Time series analysis is also used when the analytic goal is not monitoring the trend in an outcome indicator per se, but rather describing the relationship between a risk factor and the outcome. For example, in a study of the association between air pollution levels and the hospitalization rates of children with asthma, time series analysis might be used to simultaneously *control for* the overall trends in both measures; here, the impact of the trends on the hypothesized association is the primary focus, rather than the trends themselves.

With the recognition that intervention strategies are more effective as they become more targeted and specific, and as public health decision-making shifts to the local level, the context for analyzing trends is changing. The public health community is increasingly interested in examining trends for smaller populations and in smaller geographic areas. In maternal and child health, for example, describing trends in perinatal outcomes in relation to trends in prenatal care utilization within and across local service delivery areas is critical for program planning. There is also interest in examining trends in indicators of emerging health problems which, by definition, are only available for short periods of time. Describing trends in substance abuse during pregnancy or trends in antepartum medical risk factors—indicators that in most states are only available since the revision of the birth certificate in 1989—is essential for monitoring health status.

Once the focus of trend analysis is on data from small areas, small populations, or for a narrow range of time, it is necessary to draw from both the classic descriptive methods and the statistical approaches used in research studies. As numbers get smaller, for example, confidence in their accuracy is reduced and although no formal sampling has been carried out, it becomes more obvious that there is potential for error nonetheless. Reporting confidence intervals, or using other statistical methods to assess and compare trends becomes critical.

Consider the neonatal mortality rates of 3.9 and 3.0 per 1,000 live births to Native American women in 1990 in federal Regions V and VII respectively. These rates are based on 13 and 3 neonatal deaths and 3,364 and 993 live births. If, by chance, one less infant born to a Native American woman in Region V were to have died during the neonatal period, and one more infant born to a Native American woman in Region VII were to have died during the neonatal period, the neonatal mortality rates would have been 3.6 and 4.0, a reversal of the ordering seen in the observed data.

Region V

Actual Rate   Hypothetical Rate

$$\frac{13}{3,364} \times 1,000 = 3.9 \qquad \frac{12}{3,364} \times 1,000 = 3.6$$

Region VII

Actual Rate   Hypothetical Rate

$$\frac{3}{993} \times 1,000 = 3.0 \qquad \frac{4}{993} \times 1,000 = 4.0$$

The Region V and VII numbers and rates are drawn from data reported by the Midwest Maternal and Child Health Data Improvement Project (MMDIP), University of Illinois at Chicago, School of Public Health.

This illustrates how erratic rates based on small numbers can be. If the number of neonatal deaths is considered an unbiased *sample estimate*, rather than a population parameter, common statistical procedures could be used to calculate confidence limits and to test for differences between Region V and Region VII. Actually, all population numbers and rates, regardless of population size, are subject to errors of this type. When numbers are large, however, the errors are negligible and ignoring them, as has been the usual practice when presenting public health trend data, has little impact on findings and interpretation. When numbers are small, on the other hand, the impact of errors can be important.

To better understand why statistical approaches may be appropriate for trend analysis, it is useful to think of population numbers and rates as samples in time and space. For example, ten years of infant mortality data for one geographic area can be viewed as a sample taken from a multi-year, multi-area population, and as such the rates are subject to sampling error. In addition, the number of infant deaths and/or the number of live births might be slightly different in a given time or place depending on indeterminate conditions. If a year could be "sampled" repeatedly, an infant born at 11:59 on December 31st in one "sample" might be born at 12:00 on January 1st in another and thus be in the subsequent birth cohort, or an infant might survive in one "sample", but die in another since the probability of survival for an infant born with a given set of medical conditions is not fixed. These potential fluctuations may be termed *random error* as opposed to *sampling error*, but regardless, health events are seen as the result of dynamic, not fully predictable processes. (See Sampling Framework, Module 1, pages 29-32.)

Error also plays a role when trend data are available for only a short period of time since the ability to accurately characterize the overall shape of the trend is compromised by the reduced number of data points. For example, the maternal mortality rate in the U.S. has declined from slightly over 20 per 100,000 in 1970 to 7.9 per 100,000 in 1990. Most of this decrease, however, occurred prior to 1980. Since then, the rate has barely declined at all. Both the long term and the short term information are important to understanding maternal mortality. If data were only available since 1980, our view of the pattern of decrease over time in this indicator would be limited. On the other hand, future maternal mortality rates may be predicted more accurately if only the data for recent years is used since it is a fair assumption that the rates in subsequent years will be more similar to those in close proximity than to those in the more distant past. Statistical methods can be used to model trend data in various ways, incorporating appropriate assumptions about the nature of the trend in the past, present and future.

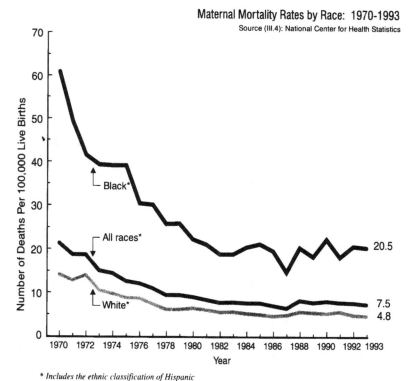

Maternal Mortality Rates by Race: 1970-1993

Source (III.4): National Center for Health Statistics

* Includes the ethnic classification of Hispanic

Reprinted from *Child Health USA '95*, U.S. Department of Health and Human Services, Public Health Service, Health Resources and Services Administration, Maternal and Child Health Bureau, DHHS Publication No. HRSA-M-DSEA-96-5.

The changing terrain of public health calls for new strategies for examining trend data. Public health professionals need guidelines for presenting trend data based on small numbers or short time periods, and principles for interpreting these types of trend data. The number of observations that give rise to the rates of interest, the extent to which the number of observations varies across populations or geographic areas to be compared, and the number of time points available for study all influence how public health agencies will analyze and report trend data.

This discussion explores conceptual and methodological issues pertaining to analyzing trend data. Advantages and disadvantages of approaches for increasing the stability of rates such as averaging data over time and / or geography, and statistical methods such as regression analysis are described. Interpretation and presentation issues are addressed throughout. Sixteen years of infant mortality data reported by the Chicago Department of Public Health are used to illustrate the analytic approaches described in the text.

WHY DO TREND ANALYSIS?

One of the hallmarks of epidemiologic analysis is the understanding that health outcomes in a population can only be fully understood if their frequency and distribution is examined in terms of person, place, and time. Trend analysis is one leg of this analytic triangle, and is used for public health surveillance and monitoring, for forecasting, for program evaluation, for policy analysis, and for etiologic analysis (investigation of potentially causal relationships between risk factors and outcomes). A study of time trends may focus, therefore, on one or more of the following:

The overall pattern of change in an indicator over time. The most general goal of trend analysis for public health surveillance is to discern whether the level of a health status, service, or systems indicator has increased or decreased over time, and if it has, how quickly or slowly the increase or decrease has occurred.

Comparing one time period to another time period. This form of trend analysis is carried out in order to assess the level of an indicator before and after an event. Evaluating the impact of programs, policy shifts, or medical and other technical advances may call for what is sometimes called interrupted time series analysis

Comparing one geographic area to another. When comparing the level of an indicator across geographic areas, only looking at one point in time can be misleading. For instance, one area may have a higher value on an indicator in one year, but a lower value in the next—analyzing the trend over several years can give a more precise comparison of the two areas.

Comparing one population to another. When comparing the level of an indicator across populations, both absolute and relative differences are important. For instance, one population may have consistently higher rates over time compared to another population and the rates in both populations may be decreasing over time, but the disparity between the rates in the two populations at each point in time may be increasing or decreasing. Analyzing the trend over time can provide information about the changing rates and the changing disparity in the rates.

Making future projections. Projecting rates into the future is a means of monitoring progress toward a national or local objective or simply providing an estimate of the rate of future occurrence. Projecting the potential number of future cases can aid in the planning of needed health and other related services and in defining corresponding resource requirements.

PREPARING TO ANALYZE TREND DATA

A series of conceptual issues must be addressed before analyzing and interpreting trend data regardless of the purpose of the analysis. These issues include:

- Sample size—the number of time periods being examined
- Presence of extreme observations or outliers
- Availability of numerator and denominator data
- Confounding—changes over time in factors related to the indicator of interest

Sample size. First, it is critical to understand the nature of the data-set being analyzed. In public health, trend analysis is typically carried out at the ecologic level. In other words, the observations, or units of analysis, are <u>time periods</u> (years, months, days) and not <u>individuals</u>. A simple data-set for use in a trend analysis might be organized in the following way:

	Year	Rate per 10,000	# of Health Events (numerator)	Population at Risk (Denominator)
1	1970	13.3	26	1,955
2	1971	12.8	24	1,877
-	-	-	-	-
-	-	-	-	-
-	-	-	-	-
-	-	-	-	-
-	-	-	-	-
25	1994	11.8	24	2,034
26	1995	12.0	26	2,164

In this hypothetical data-set, there are 26 observations, one for each year. In statistical terms, these 26 observations are a sample in time, and therefore 26 is the sample size for analysis regardless of the size of the population denominators. The fewer the number of time periods available, the smaller the sample size and as usual, the greater the potential for error. The longer the time period, the more information and therefore the more likely it is to precisely identify patterns of change. Referring again to the graph of maternal mortality shown earlier, we see that if only data from 1980 forward were examined, the lack of improvement during this time period could be misinterpreted as representing the longer term trend which, in contrast, shows considerable progress in preventing this adverse outcome.

Presence of extreme observations. Another consideration when analyzing and interpreting trends over time is whether there are extreme observations, or outliers, in the data. If there are, it is important to determine whether these are due to random variability or whether they reflect a real departure from the general trend. In the graph of the annual number of measles cases seen below, understanding the peak in 1989 and 1990 is as important as understanding the overall long term trend. In this case, the maternal and child health community used this information to focus more intensively on immunization efforts.

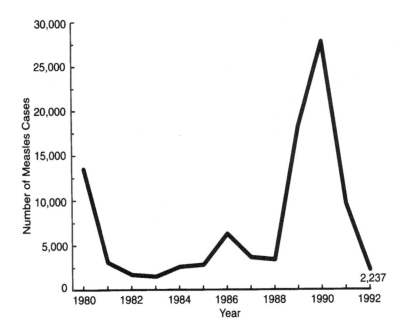

Reported Number of Measles Cases: 1980-1992

Source (III.2): Centers for Disease Control and Prevention;
Interagency Committee to Improve Access to Immunization Services:
National Vaccine Advisory Committee

Reprinted from *Child Health USA '93*, U.S. Department of Health and Human Services, Public Health Service, Health Resources and Services Administration, Maternal and Child Health Bureau, DHHS Publication No. HRSA-MCH-94-1.

Availability of numerator and denominator data. The accuracy of numerator and denominator information over time is also very important in insuring meaningful interpretation of trend data. If both numerator and denominator data for an indicator are available for each time period being studied, then these can be easily analyzed. For instance, it is relatively straightforward to examine trends in indicators based on vital records data, such as low birthweight or infant mortality, because the numerator and denominator information is collected continuously. The number of low birthweight births or the number of infant deaths as well as the total number of live births can be accurately counted on an annual or even monthly basis.

In contrast, other indicators require population denominators which are not collected continuously. Census data are collected once every 10 years, with intercensal estimates being calculated routinely only for certain geographic areas and certain populations. If a trend analysis in a small area, or comparing different age groups or sociodemographic groups is planned, it is typically quite difficult to obtain estimates for the required denominators. For example, annual estimates of the population of children less than 18 years old in a small city are probably unavailable.

When intercensal estimates are available, they have typically been calculated using what is called the Component Method. This method uses data for births, deaths, and migration patterns (in and out) in a given population to yield revised population estimates. Data from a decennial census is used as baseline data (Year 1), and then the Component Method calculates estimates for subsequent years as follows:

$$\text{Estimate}_{\text{Year 2}} = \text{Population}_{\text{Year 1}} + \text{Births}_{\text{Year 2}} \quad - \text{Deaths}_{\text{Year 2}} \quad + \text{Net Migration}_{\text{Year 2}}$$

$$\text{Estimate}_{\text{Year 3}} = \text{Population}_{\text{Year 1}} + \text{Births}_{\text{Years 2 and 3}} - \text{Deaths}_{\text{Year 2 and 3}} + \text{Net Migration}_{\text{Year 2 and 3}}$$

and so on until the final year of interest is reached.

Birth and death information is readily available for all time periods, but migration patterns are quite difficult to estimate. When the Component Method is not feasible, other approaches turn to proxy indicators of population such as school enrollment, number of filed tax returns, or car registrations to derive population estimates.

Less precise, but easiest to carry out, are simple linear interpolation or extrapolation. Linear interpolation and extrapolation both involve the calculation of average annual % change for use in estimating population denominators.

Linear Interpolation

When data are only available for the beginning and end of a time period of interest, the formula for calculating an average annual % change is as follows:

$$\text{Average Annual \% Change} = \left(\frac{\dfrac{\text{Final Value} - \text{First Value}}{\text{First Value}}}{n-1} \right) \times 100$$

$$= \left(\frac{\dfrac{\text{Final Value}}{\text{First Value}} - \dfrac{\text{First Value}}{\text{First Value}}}{n-1} \right) \times 100$$

$$= \left(\frac{\dfrac{\text{Final Value}}{\text{First Value}} - 1}{n-1} \right) \times 100$$

where n = the number of years,
inclusive of the first and final years

Suppose available census estimates of the number of children under 18 years of age in a community are:

1990	3,224
1995	3,943

The average annual percent change can then be calculated as:

$$\dfrac{\dfrac{3{,}943 - 3{,}224}{3{,}224}}{5} \times 100$$

$$= 4.46$$

Once the average percent change is calculated, it can then be applied to the baseline value, yielding a constant for use in interpolating the population values for the intervening years. In other words, to get estimates for the 4 years between the known values for 1990 and 1995, the average annual percent change of 4.46 is applied to the number of children < 18 in 1990.

$$\text{Constant} = \text{average annual \% change} \times \text{Baseline Value (1990)}$$

$$144 = 0.0446 \times 3{,}224$$

This estimate of a yearly increase of 144 children < 18 can now be added year by year to obtain new annual estimates. In general this process occurs as follows:

$$\text{Estimate}_{1991} = \text{Value}_{1990} + \text{Constant}$$

And, then again:

$$\text{Estimate}_{1992} = \text{Estimate}_{1991} + \text{Constant}$$

This process continues until the known value for 1995 is reached. For estimating the population of children under 18, we obtain:

For 1991: $3{,}368 = 3{,}224 + 144$

For 1992: $3{,}512 = 3{,}368 + 144$

For 1993: $3{,}656 = 3{,}512 + 144$

For 1994: $3{,}800 = 3{,}656 + 144$

Linear interpolation assumes that the change over time is occurring uniformly—the change from the first to the second year is the same as the change from the second to the third year, and so on. Any year to year differences are not seen, but as long as these differences can be assumed to be small, this method will yield reasonable population estimates.

Even less precise than linear interpolation, sometimes decennial census figures are used as population denominators for a whole series of years. If the populations of interest are assumed to be fairly stable, using the decennial census figures as stand-ins may be reasonable, but if the population is changing rapidly, this will result in errors and misinterpretation of trends. If this approach is taken, it is incumbent upon the analyst to describe the potential bias in the results. For example, if a single decennial census figure is used as the population denominator for each year in a five year period, but the population actually increased during that period, then any rates reported will be overestimates, and conversely, if the population actually decreased during that period, then any rates reported will be underestimates.

Confounding. Particularly when trend analysis is to be undertaken for a small area or small population, changes over time in other factors related to the indicator of interest must also be considered. For example, change in the sociodemographic characteristics of the population such as change in the age structure, the ethnic composition, or income level over time may be associated with the change over time in the indicator that is of primary interest. The question is whether comparing the health status of a community from 1970 to 1995, for example, is meaningful. Is it really the "same" community at the two endpoints of the trend analysis, or is any observed trend confounded by changes in factors other than the indicator being studied?

Changes in reporting definitions for an indicator, or reporting accuracy over time might also confound the trend information and lead to misinterpretation. For instance, varying criteria for reporting fetal deaths versus spontaneous abortions may produce spurious results when trend analysis for these indicators is carried out. Similarly, changes in medical technology which have an impact on the indicator, such as the impact on infant mortality of the widespread implementation of neonatal intensive care units in the late 1970's and early 1980's, must also be considered. Other changes over time that are of concern when conducting trend analysis include changes in laws or public policy such as a change in eligibility criteria for programs such as Medicaid, or rules concerning access to services for minors, as well as changes in cultural practices such as reduction (or increase) in substance abuse.

In general, accounting for change over time in other factors related to the indicator of interest increases in importance the longer the time period and/or the smaller the area or population size being studied. Demographic changes such as a shift in ethnic composition, for instance, may be more pronounced at the county or community level than in a state or the nation as a whole. On the other hand, a shift in cultural practices usually occurs gradually and will be identified only over a long period of time.

ANALYSIS OF TREND DATA

The selection of a strategy for analyzing trend data will depend in part on the purpose of the analysis, and on careful consideration of all of the issues discussed above. Once there is a sound conceptual framework, tables, graphs and statistical analysis are tools for examining and analyzing trend data; graphs, in particular, are an effective tool for presenting the pattern of change over time.

Regardless of whether statistical techniques will be used for analyzing data over time, the most straightforward and intuitive first step in assessing a trend is to plot the actual observed numbers or rates of interest by year (or some other time period deemed appropriate). In addition, the numbers or rates should be examined in tabular form.

These initial steps are indispensable for understanding the general shape of the trend, for identifying any outliers in the data, and for becoming familiar with both the absolute and relative levels of the numbers and rates being studied. Inspection of the data provides the basis for making subsequent analysis choices and should never be bypassed.

Visual inspection of the data may indicate that use of statistical procedures is inappropriate. For example, an outlier at a particular point in time may be of intrinsic interest, representing circumstances in the community important to understand. Statistical procedures, such as regression analysis, would mute the effect of this outlier by assuming that its extreme value is attributable to statistical instability. For example, a sudden rise in the rate of injury deaths due to drowning may point to a problem at community swimming facilities and it would be unfortunate and inappropriate if a statistical examination of an overall trend were to obscure this information.

Visual inspection also permits a preliminary assessment of the overall direction and shape of the trend. Commonly used statistical approaches are designed for assessing *linear* trends; that is, a series of numbers or rates which change over time in a consistent, or uniform, fashion. If the trend appears to be different during distinct time periods, either in shape or direction, then an analytic method must be selected that will preserve and not obscure this important information.

In addition, when the number of health events is very small, individual case review may be called for rather than the application of statistical methods. Each event might appropriately be considered as a sentinel or unexpected occurrence, arising from different processes than when health events occur on a widespread basis.

In order to look more concretely at the process of analyzing trends, data reported by the Chicago Department of Public Health are used throughout the remainder of this discussion. The data presented here are for what is referred to as Chicago Community Area 33, representing a small area of the city. Chicago Community Area 33 is an aggregation of five census tracts. As recommended, we first look at the actual data, both in tabular and graphic form:

Infant Mortality Rates
Chicago Community Area 33 1979-1994

	Deaths	Births	Rate / 1,000	95% CI*
1979	8	213	37.6	11.6-63.6
1980	7	220	31.8	8.2-55.4
1981	6	179	33.5	6.7-60.3
1982	7	202	34.7	9.0-60.4
1983	5	172	29.1	3.6-54.6
1984	8	184	43.5	13.4-73.6
1985	4	183	21.9	0.5-43.3
1986	4	189	21.2	0.4-42.0
1987	7	194	36.1	9.4-62.8
1988	5	181	27.6	3.4-51.8
1989	9	227	39.6	13.7-65.5
1990	6	252	23.8	4.8-42.8
1991	4	247	16.2	0.3-32.1
1992	3	246	12.2	0.0-26.0
1993	10	244	41.0	15.6-66.4
1994	6	275	21.8	4.3-39.3

$$* \, 95\% \text{ Confidence Interval (CI)} = \text{Rate} \pm 1.96 \sqrt{\frac{\text{rate}}{\text{pop}}} \times 1,000$$

$$\text{For example, for 1994, the 95\% CI} = 21.8 \pm 1.96 \sqrt{\frac{21.8}{275}} \times 1,000$$

$$= 21.8 \pm 1.96 \times 8.9$$

$$= 21.8 \pm 17.5$$

$$= 4.3 - 39.3$$

Infant Mortality

Observed Rates by Year
Chicago Community Area 33

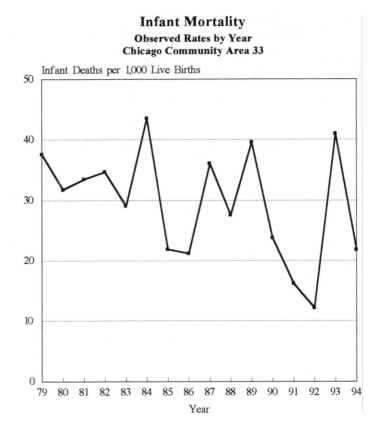

Infant Mortality

Observed Rates and Confidence Limits by Year
Chicago Community Area 33

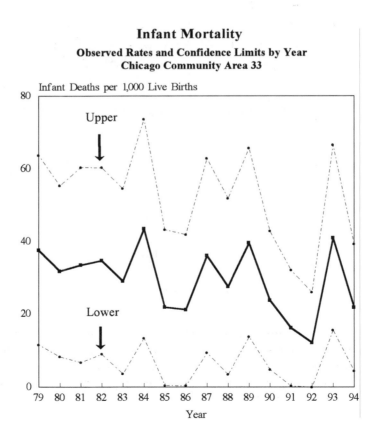

These preliminary views of the community area infant mortality data show a series of unstable rates—the confidence intervals around each rate are very wide and the pattern over time is quite jagged. Ten or fewer infant deaths and fewer than 300 live births occur each year in this area. Due to this instability, it is very difficult to meaningfully interpret the data and other techniques have to be applied in order to create a clearer picture of the pattern over time. (Note that the Y axis scaling on the two graphs is different; the scale on the second graph had to be expanded in order to accommodate the wide confidence limits.)

Data Transformation and Smoothing

One step toward improving the interpretability of the data is to put the rates on a logarithmic scale. A log transformation of the data provides more appropriate and realistic results because it "flattens" the series of rates. While the overall shape of the trend is unchanged, the rate of increase or decrease is somewhat altered. For example, if rates are decreasing over time and no transformation is carried out, future projections will eventually predict the occurrence of zero health events, but the log transformation will slow the approach to zero (and in fact never reach zero) making any projection of future rates more reasonable.

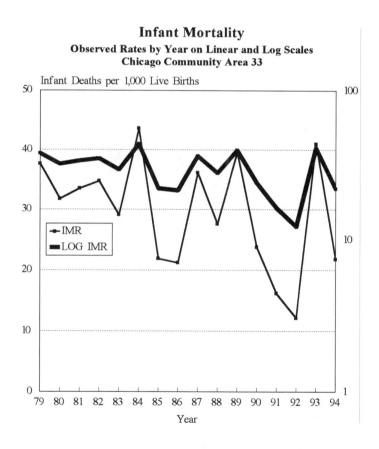

Next, if the initial assessment does not reveal any outliers in the data, more elaborate statistical methods beyond simple transformation of the rates may be worthwhile. In general, statistical approaches aim to "smooth" the data; that is, they aim to increase the stability of the rates and hence diminish their jagged appearance. Various forms of averaging, including use of multiple year rates, moving averages, and regression procedures can accomplish the desired smoothing.

Perhaps the form of averaging most commonly carried out by MCH and other public health professionals is collapsing data across time periods—for instance, calculating rates by combining the numerators and denominators for two or three years of data rather than using the annual rates. This approach increases the stability of the resulting rates by increasing the sample size at each time point. The infant mortality rate for 1979-1980 in Chicago Community Area 33 is:

$$\frac{8+7}{213+220} \times 1{,}000 = \frac{15}{433} \times 1{,}000 = 34.6$$

Collapsing data in this fashion, however, though it increases stability, also means a loss of information. With 16 years of data, for example, using two year rates leaves only 8 data points to portray the pattern over time. If more years of data were combined, the loss of information would render it difficult to discern any pattern. Below is a plot of the infant mortality data for Chicago Community Area 33 using two year rates.

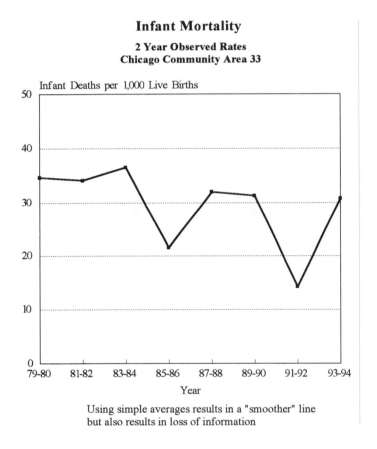

Infant Mortality

2 Year Observed Rates
Chicago Community Area 33

Using simple averages results in a "smoother" line
but also results in loss of information

Moving averages are also used to increase stability and "smooth" the data. Here, time periods are not combined in mutually exclusive groups as when simple multiple year rates are calculated, but rather in overlapping sequences:

>Years 1,2, and 3
>Years 2,3, and 4
>Years 3,4, and 5
>etc. until the last year is included

Moving averages have the advantage of increasing stability with a minimal loss of information. Compared with the 8 data points resulting from calculation of two year mutually exclusive rates as shown above, 15 data points result from calculation of rates based on two year moving averages. The maintenance of information with moving averages makes it possible to combine more years of data to maximize sample size at each point. For instance, calculation of three year moving averages with the 16 years of data results in only 2 data points being lost, leaving 14 to portray the pattern over time. Below is a plot of the infant mortality data for Chicago Community Area 33 using three year moving averages.

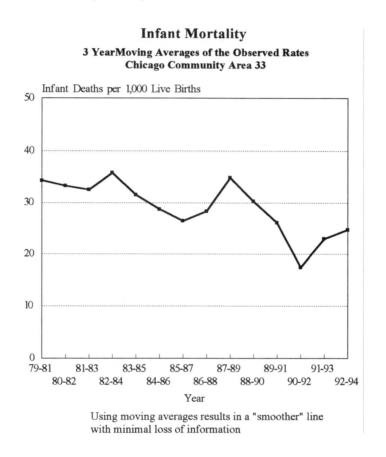

Infant Mortality

3 YearMoving Averages of the Observed Rates
Chicago Community Area 33

Using moving averages results in a "smoother" line
with minimal loss of information

Reporting Average Annual Percent Change in an Indicator

Earlier, average annual percent change was discussed in the context of linear interpolation when estimates of population denominators were required in order to assemble reasonable trend data. Using average annual percent change after the trend data has been assembled and organized is somewhat different. Here, there is information on the year to year changes rather than just the overall change from the beginning to the end of a time period and the goal is to estimate how fast or slow change is occurring. The formula for average annual % change in this context is:

$$\frac{\left(\sum_{i=2}^{n} \dfrac{\text{Rate}_{\text{Year i}}}{\text{Rate}_{\text{Year i-1}}} - 1\right) \times 100}{n-1}$$

where n is the total number of years

Year 1 is the first year

Year n is the final year

If numbers or rates are unstable and therefore the pattern very jagged, the average of the year to year changes if no preliminary smoothing is carried out can be misleading. For example, the average of the observed set of 15 annual % changes for the 16 infant mortality rates in Community Area 33 is calculated as:

$$\frac{\left[\left(\dfrac{31.8}{37.6}-1\right)+\left(\dfrac{33.5}{31.8}-1\right)+\ldots+\left(\dfrac{41.0}{12.1}-1\right)+\left(\dfrac{21.8}{41.0}-1\right)\right] \times 100}{15} = 10.5$$

The result of 10.5 % implies that the infant mortality rates are increasing over time, a result which contradicts the pattern of decreasing rates over time seen in the plots shown earlier.

Using the 13 three year moving averages to gain stability and smoothness, however, the average annual % change is:

$$\frac{\left[\left(\dfrac{33.3}{34.3}-1\right)+\left(\dfrac{32.5}{33.3}-1\right)+\ldots+\left(\dfrac{23.1}{17.4}-1\right)+\left(\dfrac{24.8}{23.1}-1\right)\right] \times 100}{13} = -1.1$$

This implies that the infant mortality rates are decreasing by approximately 1.1 %, a result much more consistent with what is seen in the plots of the data.

Average annual percent change can also be used to calculate a projected rate. This is accomplished through linear extrapolation, by iteratively increasing or decreasing the number or rate according to the average annual percent change. For the infant mortality rates based on 3 year moving averages in Community Area 33, the process would be as follows:

$$\text{Projected Rate}_{93\text{-}94\text{-}95} = \text{Observed Rate}_{92\text{-}93\text{-}94} + (-0.011 \times \text{Observed Rate}_{92\text{-}93\text{-}94})$$

And, then again:

$$\text{Projected Rate}_{94\text{-}95\text{-}96} = \text{Projected Rate}_{93\text{-}94\text{-}95} + (-0.011 \times \text{Projected Rate}_{93\text{-}94\text{-}95})$$

And this would continue for as many years as considered appropriate. For Community Area 33, the first two projected rates are:

$$\text{Projected Rate}_{93\text{-}94\text{-}95} : 24.5 = 24.8 + \left(-0.011 \times 24.8\right)$$

$$\text{Projected Rate}_{94\text{-}95\text{-}96} : 24.2 = 24.5 + \left(-0.011 \times 24.5\right)$$

And if this process of linear extrapolation were continued, the projected infant mortality rate for the three year period 1999-2000-2001 would be 22.7.

In order to calculate a confidence limit around a projected rate arrived at in this fashion, the average annual % change in the population denominator has to be computed and then linear extrapolation used to obtain an estimate for the projected year of interest. For the infant mortality data, for instance, the average annual percent change in total live births (or the average change in the 3 year moving total live births) would be calculated and then applied iteratively into the future. A 95 % confidence interval can then be generated with the usual formula:

$$\text{Projected Rate} \pm 1.96 \sqrt{\frac{\text{Projected Rate}}{\text{Projected Live Births}} \times 1000}$$

Comment

Technically, the above formula is not quite correct because the projected live births in the denominator is also an estimated quantity rather than a fixed number (such as the known number of live births used when analyzing current data); the resulting confidence interval will be an underestimate (narrower) than if a more complex formula were used.

Statistical Procedures

In order to test whether there is a statistically significant trend or whether two or more trends are statistically different, several approaches are available. In contrast to the averaging and smoothing techniques discussed so far, statistical analysis has the advantage of jointly considering the information contained in the series of counts or rates, rather than considering each time point separately. Analyzing the original series of rates as a unit in effect imposes stability without other transformations of the data.

Chi-Square Test for Linear Trend

A chi-square test for trend can be obtained by organizing the observed data into a contingency table with one row for each time period and two columns: the first for the number of individuals who experienced the health outcome (the numerator of the rate); the second for the number of individuals who did not (the denominator minus the numerator). Following is modified output from Epi-Info showing the chi-square test for trend for the 16 annual infant mortality rates in Chicago Community Area 33:

Analysis For Linear Trend In Proportions

Exposure Score	Cases	Controls
1979.00	8.00	205.00
1980.00	7.00	213.00
1981.00	6.00	173.00
1982.00	7.00	195.00
1983.00	5.00	167.00
1984.00	8.00	176.00
1985.00	4.00	179.00
1986.00	4.00	185.00
1987.00	7.00	187.00
1988.00	8.00	176.00
1989.00	9.00	218.00
1990.00	6.00	247.00
1991.00	4.00	243.00
1992.00	3.00	243.00
1993.00	10.00	234.00
1994.00	6.00	269.00

Chi Square for linear trend : 1.583   p value : 0.20838

The linear trend in these data is not statistically significant according to this test since the p-value is 0.2, not less than the customary cutoff of 0.05.

Regression Analysis

As an outgrowth of jointly considering the whole series of counts or rates, regression procedures also generate a complementary series of predicted counts or rates. A confidence band around this set of predicted values can be calculated, and will be narrower than the confidence limits calculated around each count or rate separately, reflecting the smoothing implicitly carried out by the regression procedure. (*See the Technical Notes at the end of the module.*)

In addition, regression procedures will generate estimates of future rates as well as estimates of average annual percent change, neither of which are automatically obtained when averaging without modeling is carried out or when a contingency table is organized to conduct a chi-square test for trend. Moreover, graphs of the predicted and projected values as well as the confidence band can be plotted.

Another advantage of using regression methods for analyzing trends and making projections is that other variables can be included in a model. For instance, if annual infant mortality rates are to be modeled, annual data on rates of prenatal care utilization, or rates of substance abuse during pregnancy, or changes in demographic risk markers could be simultaneously examined. With trend data, regression procedures model the association between time and the outcome of interest; if other variables are confounders or effect modifiers of this association, the predicted rates, the projected rates, and the confidence bands around these will be adjusted appropriately. Without using some form of regression modeling, the impact of other variables cannot be accounted for in the results.

There are several regression approaches that can be employed to examine trend data. Following is a generic description of these approaches.

Ordinary Least Squares (OLS) Regression

Ordinary least squares (OLS) regression can be used to model the observed series of rates, but as stated above, it is often preferable to model the natural logarithm of the rates. The disparity between predicted rates based on linear and log linear models increases as the time periods being forecasted move further from the time of observation. Multiple year rates or moving averages (or the log transformation of these) may also be modeled using the OLS method. A simple OLS model has the general form:

For modeling the actual rates

$$rate_i = Intercept + (Slope \times Year_i)$$

For modeling the natural logarithm of the rates:

$$\ln(rate_i) = Intercept + (Slope \times Year_i)$$

where i = 1 to the number of years being analyzed

The figure below again shows the observed rates for Chicago Community Area 33 along with both the predicted values (regression line) obtained from modeling the actual rates and the predicted values (regression line) obtained from modeling the natural logarithm of the rates. You can see that the regression line from modeling the actual rates crosses the regression line from modeling the transformed rates in approximately the year 2006. If the line for the actual rates is used, the infant mortality rate is predicted to be zero by the year 2023, whereas it is predicted to be approximately 8 per 1,000 live births in that same year if the regression line from the log transformed rates is used. In fact, using the log transformation, an infant mortality rate of zero will never be predicted, which unfortunately, is a more realistic result.

Infant Mortality
Observed Rates by Year
and Linear and Log Linear Regression Lines
Chicago Community Area 33

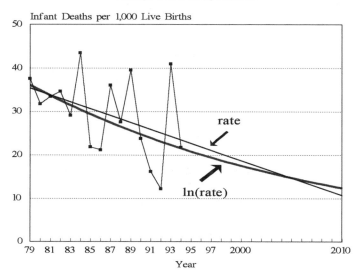

From the point of view of an OLS regression procedure, the sample size equals the number of time points being modeled. The procedure does not have access to information on the populations sizes that gave rise to the rates at each time point. In other words, OLS regression accounts for the variability across time periods, but cannot account for the variability or random error in each individual rate.

When modeling the 16 years of Chicago data with OLS, then, the sample size equals 16 regardless of whether the population (in this case, live births) in the denominator of each rate is in the 100s, 1,000s, or 100,000s. The confidence band around the OLS regression line will therefore be identical for sets of the same rates even if these arise from populations of different size. For example, if another community area in Chicago had exactly the same set of rates as those for Community Area 33, but these were based on many more live births each year, OLS regression would not distinguish between the two areas.

To illustrate, suppose that the 1994 rate of 21.8 in another community area was based on 27,500 rather than on 275 live births. The OLS procedure would not recognize this difference; the sample size remains 16, and the regression lines, the confidence bands, and other statistics such as average annual percent change would be identical. This is despite the fact that there is much less potential for error in the set of more stable rates compared with the set of unstable ones.

Further, if two year rates were modeled in order to gain stability, the sample size would be reduced from 16 to only 8 data points. While the confidence band around the line would be narrower as a result of the smoothing, there would be loss of statistical power due to the smaller sample size. Again, modeling moving averages has the advantage of both increasing stability and maintaining sample size. Below is the plot of the ordinary least square regression results of modeling the natural logarithm of the 3 year moving averages for Chicago Community Area 33.

Infant Mortality
3 Year Moving Averages, Regression Line and Confidence Band
Modeling the Natural Log Transformation
Chicago Community Area 33

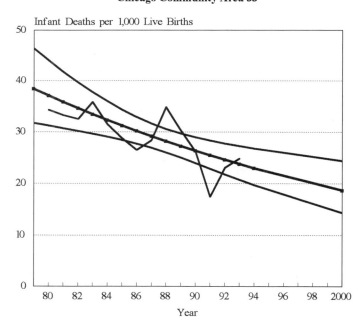

Poisson Regression

Poisson regression can also be used to model the observed rates, collapsed data, or moving averages. Because of the nature of the Poisson distribution, by definition a log transformation of the data is employed.

In contrast to ordinary least squares regression, Poisson regression has the advantage of accounting both for the fluctuation across time and the variability at each time point. The procedure models the actual number of health events (numerator) given the total population at risk (denominator) at each time point rather than the pre-calculated rates. In essence, this approach is equivalent to having data at the individual level, with sample size equaling the number of *individuals* in the denominators of the rates instead of the number of *time points* for which rates are available.

For example, a Poisson regression procedure will model the 6 infant deaths given the 275 births that occurred in Chicago Community Area 33 in 1994 or the 600 infant deaths given the 27,500 live births that occurred in some hypothetical community area, rather than modeling the rate representation of 21.8 for both areas as is done in OLS. The confidence band around a Poisson regression line, therefore, will be different for sets of the same rates when they arise from populations of different size. A simple Poisson model has the general form:

$$\ln\left(\frac{\#\text{ of health events}_i}{\#\text{ in population at risk}_i}\right) = \text{Intercept} + (\text{Slope} \times \text{Year}_i)$$

where $i = 1$ to the number of years being analyzed

Despite the differences between the OLS and Poisson procedures, in most circumstances the results from using OLS to model the natural logarithm of rates or Poisson regression will be quite similar. Understanding when and how these two regression procedures might differ, however, is important for choosing an appropriate method to use.

When a set of rates is based on small numbers, the variability of each rate is large, and the variability across time will probably also be large (a jagged pattern). In this scenario, the confidence band from either Poisson or OLS regression will be wide since both the small numbers and the jagged pattern over time imply instability. The confidence band from Poisson regression will be somewhat wider because it incorporates information about both kinds of variability, while OLS only incorporates information about the variability across time, but the difference will not be great.

On the other hand, in the improbable scenario that a set of rates based on small numbers shows little variability across time (a smooth pattern), the confidence band from Poisson regression will be quite a bit wider than that from OLS. Here, the small numbers and the smooth pattern carry contradictory information about stability. Poisson regression calculates a confidence band based on both pieces of information, but places heavier weight on the population sizes with, in this case, their implication of instability, while OLS regression calculates a narrower confidence band based solely on the smooth pattern over time with its implication of stability.

When a set of rates is based on large numbers, the variability of each rate is small, and the variability across time will probably also be small (smooth pattern). In this scenario, the confidence band from either Poisson or OLS regression will be narrow since both the large numbers and the smooth pattern over time imply stability. In fact, the confidence bands will be almost identical because the variability of each rate is very close to zero.

On the other hand, in the improbable scenario that a set of rates based on large numbers shows a lot of variability across time (jagged pattern), the confidence band from Poisson regression will be quite a bit narrower than that from OLS. Now the large numbers and the jagged pattern carry contradictory information about stability. Poisson regression calculates a confidence band based on both pieces of information, but again places heavier weight on the population sizes with, in this case, their implication of stability, while OLS regression calculates a wider confidence band based solely on the jagged pattern over time with its implication of instability.

Because it is much more likely that the variability across time and the variability in the rates are consistent with each other, rather than contradictory, the results from Poisson and OLS regression will usually yield similar results. Often, in public health agencies, OLS regression is used because this procedure is available in many different software packages, whereas Poisson regression is available only in more specialized software.

Time Series Analysis

Time Series Analysis refers to a collection of specialized regression methods that use integrated moving averages and other smoothing techniques and have different assumptions about the error structure of the data. The term "moving average" as used in time series analysis should not be confused with the calculation of moving averages as has been demonstrated above. Here, the term refers to a complex process that incorporates information from past observations and past errors in those observations into the estimation of predicted values.

Unlike ordinary least squares, logistic or Poisson regression which assume that errors in the modeled observations are independent (uncorrelated), time series methods assume that the errors are correlated. Time series methods can diagnose the precise nature of the correlation and adjust for it. In general, correlation in the errors increases the variance of the regression estimates, and therefore using these methods will yield wider confidence bands than the other approaches already discussed. The regression estimates themselves will also be somewhat different, and despite the wider confidence band, the efficiency of time series methods may result in a steeper slope than that generated by OLS or Poisson regression.

In many public health data-sets, the extent of correlation in the errors is not always high. If possible, statistical software such as SAS should be used to diagnose whether correlated errors are a significant problem. If they are not, then OLS or Poisson regression can be used without seriously violating the assumption of independence inherent in these approaches.

There are many other features of time series methods that aid in precisely characterizing a trend, including identification and adjustment for non-linear components of the trend and differential weighting of observations for forecasting. While time series methods yield more precise results, their use also requires specialized software and more advanced technical expertise, and therefore, building them into routine surveillance and monitoring activities is rarely feasible. If these methods are to be used, the assistance of a statistician should be sought.

Results of Regression Analysis

The following table provides a comparison of the results obtained from using various regression approaches to model the sixteen years of infant mortality data for Chicago Community Area 33. For simplicity, only the results for 1994 are shown. The OLS and Poisson results shown are quite similar. The time series approach yields a similar predicted value, but a wider confidence band as expected. Despite the differences, these approaches will probably not lead to different public health conclusions.

Estimated Infant Mortality Rates and 95% Confidence Bands
Various Regression Approaches
Chicago Community Area 33

Method	1994
OLS Regression, Modeling the Natural Logarithm of the Rates	21.5 15.4-30.2
Poisson Regression	23.7 16.4-34.2
Time Series Analysis—the AR(1) Model Using the Natural Logarithm of the Rates	19.6 8.9-43.2

An estimate of average annual % change and projected rates can be obtained directly from the output of a regression procedure rather than having to conduct the iterative calculations demonstrated earlier. The following are regression results generated by SAS® for modeling the natural logarithm of the 16 infant mortality rates for Chicago Community Area 33:

```
ANNUAL IM RATES FOR CHICAGO COMMUNITY AREAS

AREA=33

Model: MODEL1
Dependent Variable: LNIMRATE

Analysis of Variance

                        Sum of          Mean
Source          DF      Squares         Square      F Value      Prob>F

Model           1       0.40427         0.40427     3.722        0.0742
Error           14      1.52046         0.10860
C Total         15      1.92472

        Root MSE        0.32955     R-square    0.2100
        Dep Mean        3.32866     Adj R-sq    0.1536
        C.V.            9.90043

Parameter Estimates

                    Parameter       Standard     T for H0:
Variable    DF      Estimate        Error        Parameter=0      Prob > ]T]

INTERCEP    1       6.311364        1.54815934   4.077            0.0011
YEAR        1       -0.034482       0.01787243   -1.929           0.0742
```

As was seen in the table comparing different regression approaches, the predicted value for 1994 using OLS regression to model the natural logarithm of the infant mortality rates is:

$$e^{a+b \times \text{YEAR}}$$

$$e^{6.311+(-0.0345 \times 94)} = 21.5$$

Remember that because the natural logarithm of the infant mortality rates were modeled, the regression estimates need to be exponentiated in order to report the results in the usual units.

The average annual percent change based on the predicted values from the log linear regression analysis is:

$$(e^{-0.0345} - 1) \times 100 = -3.4$$

This formula is exactly the same as the one used before when the calculation for average annual percent change was carried out iteratively with the observed data—here the beta coefficient (slope or parameter estimate) from the regression results is the ratio of the rate in one year to the rate in the previous year (the relative risk). This is seen more clearly if the formula is written as follows:

$$\left(\frac{e^{6.311+(-0.0345 \times 94)}}{e^{6.311+(-0.0345 \times 93)}} - 1 \right) \times 100$$

$$= \left(e^{-0.0345 \times (94-93)} - 1 \right) \times 100$$

$$= \left(e^{-0.0345} - 1 \right) \times 100$$

$$= -3.4$$

Notice that modeling the 16 annual log transformed rates, the average annual % change is negative, indicating a decreasing infant mortality rate. This is in contrast to the result obtained earlier when the average annual percent change was computed without any modeling or smoothing. Without modeling, moving averages had to be used in order to generate a reasonable result, but here the regression procedure itself accomplished the necessary smoothing. Of note is that the regression estimate of a 3.4% annual decrease in infant mortality is quite a bit higher than the estimate of a 1.1 % annual decrease obtained earlier when using the 3 year moving averages without any modeling. This result reflects the use of the predicted rather than the actual values in the calculation.

Using the results of regression analysis, projected rates can also be calculated directly from the regression equation. The calculation is the same as for any predicted value, except that the time period of interest is outside the range of the observed data. Following are 2 projected rates using the log linear regression results:

The projected rate for 1995 : $e^{6.311+(-0.0345 \times 95)} = 20.8$

The projected rate for 2000 : $e^{6.311+(-0.0345 \times 100)} = 17.5$

Consistent with its higher estimate of average annual percent change, the regression projected rate of 17.5 for the year 2000 is lower than the projected rate of 22.7 calculated earlier for the year 2000 when using the 3 year moving averages without any modeling.

OTHER CONSIDERATIONS WHEN SELECTING GRAPHING OR STATISTICAL APPROACHES

Whether only one series of rates or multiple series of rates are being analyzed. The choice of how many years, if any, to combine when calculating moving averages may change. It may be determined that 3 year moving averages are appropriate for analyzing data from a particular geographic area. Another area, however, may require the use of 4 year moving averages in order to achieve adequate smoothing. If the two areas are to be compared, the same amount of averaging should be applied to both.

If Chicago data were to be analyzed for the city as a whole, no averaging at all would be necessary since the stability of the city rates yields a smooth pattern. If, however, a comparison were to be made between the city and one or more community areas with their jagged patterns, then averaging would have to be applied to all of the data, and applied in a comparable fashion. Below are three plots of the infant mortality rates in Chicago Community Area 33, Chicago Community Area 35, and the city as a whole. The first examines the three sets of annual observed rates:

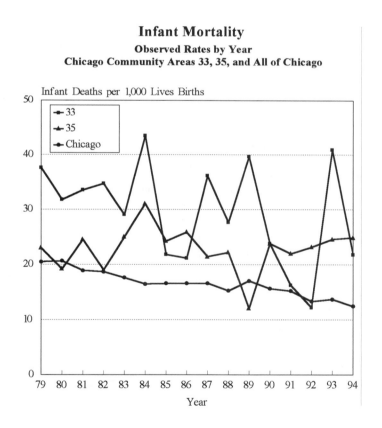

The second plot examines the three sets of 3 year moving averages, and the third the predicted values from modeling the natural logarithm of these using ordinary least squares regression:

Infant Mortality

3 Year Moving Averages of the Observed Rates by Year
Chicago Community Areas 33, 35, and All of Chicago

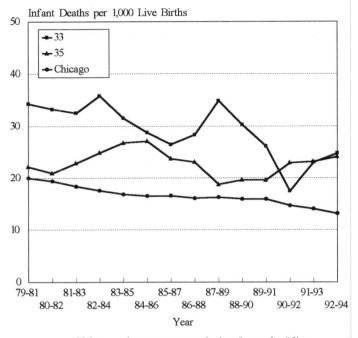

Using moving averages results in a "smoother" line
with minimal loss of information

Infant Mortality

Regession Lines
Modeling the Natural Log of the 3 Year Moving Averages
Chicago Community Areas 33, 35, and All of Chicago

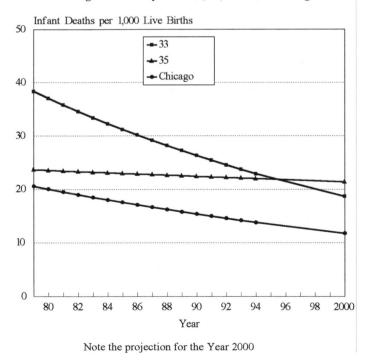

Note the projection for the Year 2000

The first plot is difficult to interpret since there is so much fluctuation in the rates in the two community areas. The comparison between the city and the two community areas is easier to see in the second and third plots. It appears that Community Area 33 has generally had a higher infant mortality rate than Community Area 35, although, particularly in the plot of the regression analysis, it appears that the rate is decreasing faster in Community Area 33.

Characteristics of other independent variables to be included in a regression model. It might be desirable to build a more complicated regression model that would include several independent variables in addition to the time variable. Inclusion of other variables can yield a more precise picture of a trend by accounting for changes over time in other factors. A model of this type might look like:

$$\ln(\text{rate}_i) = \text{intercept} + (\text{slope}_1 \times \text{Year}_i) + (\text{slope}_2 \times \text{Var1}_i) + (\text{slope}_3 \times \text{Var2}_i)$$

Remember that trend analysis is generally carried out using aggregate data. Independent variables in the model, therefore, are typically proportions and not values for individuals. For example, a model might include the annual percent of poverty in a community or the percent of women who did not receive prenatal care in a community.

Sometimes there are as many data points for these other variables as there are for the rates of the outcome being modeled; sometimes, however, there are fewer data points. For example, with 16 years of data, there may be only 2 census values available for another variable of interest. In addition, an independent variable may also need to be transformed, for instance, to the log scale prior to analysis. Moreover, in epidemiologic terms, time is the "exposure" variable in trend analysis, and therefore another variable must be related to both time and the outcome being studied in order to be a confounder of the association between these two (the trend). To be an effect modifier, the rate of change in the outcome over time (the slope of the trend) must be different at each level of another variable.

Achieving stability by combining geographic areas. In addition to or instead of smoothing trend data by using multiple year rates or moving averages, geographic areas can be combined to gain stability. As with any averaging technique, there is loss of information when areas are combined, but if the areas are similar with respect to the characteristics of their residents and/or the characteristics of their health service delivery systems, this is a viable approach.

Combining geographic areas can reduce the data burden when many comparisons are of interest, and can provide a more concise picture of the trend in a health indicator. Further, areas may be combined in a way that is most informative for health assessment, planning, and evaluation. Below are two plots of the infant mortality rates in Chicago Community Areas 33 and 35 combined, and the city as a whole. Although these two areas showed somewhat different trends in infant mortality as seen in the previous graphs, they are very similar demographically, and combining them may make more sense from the standpoint of intervention strategies. The first plot examines the 3 year moving averages of the observed rates, and the second examines the regression lines and confidence bands from modeling the natural logarithm of these.

Infant Mortality

3 Year Moving Averages of the Observed Rates by Year
Chicago Community Areas 33 & 35 combined, and Chicago

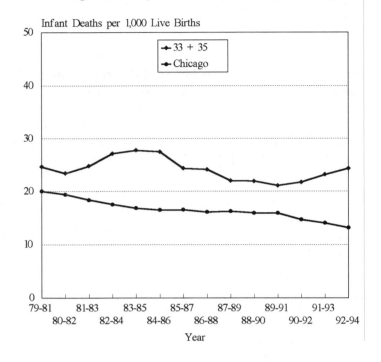

Infant Mortality

Regression Lines and Confidence Bands
Modeling the Natural Logarithm of the 3 YearMoving Averages
Chicago Community Areas 33 & 35 combined, and Chicago

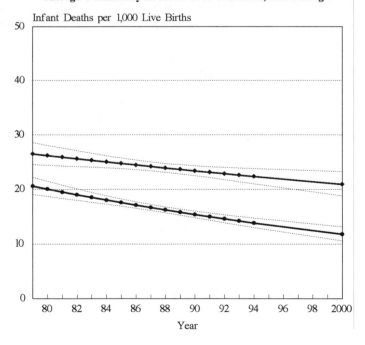

Comment

Although regression results based on moving averages have been shown here for purposes of illustration, it is more typical to use moving averages to achieve smoothing when plotting the observed data, but to use the original series of rates when conducting regression analysis. This is because, as we've seen, the regression procedure itself accomplishes the desired smoothing, and in addition, modeling moving averages may exacerbate the problem of potentially correleated data points.

TREND ANALYSIS AND USE OF LOCAL, STATE, OR NATIONAL OBJECTIVES

Using trend data, several indicators can be projected out to the point at which each meets or surpasses the appropriate Year 2000 Objective (or any other objective), and then a comparison across these indicators can be made according to the number of years behind or ahead of the objective. For example, suppose trend analysis yielded the following projections for three indicators:

- Indicator #1 — 2004
- Indicator #2 — 1999
- Indicator #3 — 2003

In this scenario, priority might be given to improving indicator #1 (assuming other factors have been taken into account) since it appears to be farther from its Year 2000 Objective than the other two indicators.

In addition, statistical testing can be carried out to assess the current level of indicators with respect to the appropriate Year 2000 (or other) Objective. The resulting z-tests can then be compared across indicators. The formula for a z-test, using an objective as a standard is as follows:

$$z_1 = \frac{\text{Indicator}_{1\,current} - \text{Objective}_1}{\sqrt{\dfrac{\text{Objective}_1}{n_{1\,current}} \times \text{multiplier}}}$$

$$z_2 = \frac{\text{Indicator}_{2\,current} - \text{Objective}_2}{\sqrt{\dfrac{\text{Objective}_2}{n_{2\,current}} \times \text{multiplier}}}$$

where n_1 and n_2 are the population denominators
giving rise to Indicator$_1$ and Indicator$_2$ respectively

Further, z-tests can be generated using projected levels of the indicators instead of the current levels. Comparisons can then be made across indicators according to these scores:

$$z_1 = \frac{\text{Indicator}_{1\,\text{projected}} - \text{Objective}_1}{\sqrt{\dfrac{\text{Objective}_1}{n_{1\,\text{projected}}} \times \text{multiplier}}}$$

$$z_2 = \frac{\text{Indicator}_{2\,\text{projected}} - \text{Objective}_2}{\sqrt{\dfrac{\text{Objective}_2}{n_{2\,\text{projected}}} \times \text{multiplier}}}$$

where n_1 and n_2 are the population denominators
giving rise to Indicator$_1$ and Indicator$_2$ respectively

Comment

Earlier we saw that the usual formula for calculating a confidence interval around a rate will yield too narrow a result (an underestimate) when a projected, rather than a known number is in the denominator of the standard error. Analogously, when a comparing a projected indicator with an objective, the result will be too large (an overestimate) since the underestimate of the standard error leads to a larger value for the z-test.

The results of using the current level of the indicator and the projected level of the indicator may yield different, but equally important information. One indicator may currently be farther from an objective than another indicator, but it may also be exhibiting a faster rate of decline over time and therefore be projected to be closer to its objective than the other indicator at some point in the future. These types of analyses can complement the information obtained from examining plots of trend data, comparing average annual percent changes or other statistical results.

PRESENTATION OF TREND DATA

The discussion thus far has described a range of analytic methods useful for understanding and interpreting trend data. Deciding which results to present and the form in which to present them is an important aspect of turning the data into information. As a general rule, it is important that public health analysts within a health agency carry out as refined and as detailed an analysis as is feasible, even though the final reports or forums for presenting the information may incorporate only portions, sometimes only small portions, of the work. Examining the data in multiple and varied forms allows for exploration of different presentation strategies, and is necessary for selecting an effective and useful approach. If analytic shortcuts are taken, this process cannot occur and the final product may suffer.

For instance, initial analysis may explore approaches to combining years or geographic areas. One averaging method may obscure an important trend, another may highlight it; unless the preliminary work is carried out, inappropriate choices for presentation may be made. In addition, having multiple analyses provides a pool from which to draw depending on the audience and circumstances of the presentation. If time and resources permit, then, the following analyses should be conducted for internal use:

1. Produce plots of the observed data along with confidence limits
2. Produce tables of the observed data along with confidence limits
3. Assess whether there are extreme observations, or outliers, in the data
4. Consider case review if numbers of events are very small
5. Consider transforming the data to a logarithmic scale
6. Assess whether the trend is linear or whether its shape or direction changes over time
7. Consider examining trends separately for subsets of the population
8. If data are based on small numbers, explore different smoothing strategies:
   a. Combine multiple years of data into mutually exclusive groups
   b. Combine multiple years of data into moving averages
   c. Combine geographic areas
9. Calculate average percent change, either annual or some other time increment
10. Calculate projected rates, particularly with respect to relevant health objectives
11. Use statistical testing, such as the chi-square test for trend or regression analysis
12. Explore different formulations for regression modeling
    a. Produce plots of the predicted and projected values, and confidence bands
    b. Explore the impact on the trend of including other variables in a model
    c. Calculate average percent change, either annual or some other time increment

Once the above analyses are generated, the following are general guidelines for presentation to a wider audience:

At Minimum	Optional
Display plots of the observed data over time	Display a table of the rates along with confidence limits
Comment in narrative form on the stability of the rates and approaches used to increase it	Display plots of predicted and projected values from regression analysis
Report average percent change	Overlay plots for different populations or geographic areas
Using narrative, interpret the relationship of the trend to reaching health status objectives, to health services utilization, and to systems functioning	Report the results of statistical testing, either for one trend or for comparisons across populations or geographic areas

Although the observed data, if based on small numbers, may be very hard to interpret due to a jagged pattern over time, most audiences need to see the original "real" numbers or rates before they can understand transformed data or regression results. For example, a community group may wish to see data for its area alone, even though a clearer picture might be obtained if data for several communities were combined. Often, it is decided not to show plots of regression results, but to simply report some of the information that a regression analysis yields such as an average percent change or a prediction of a future rate.

SUMMARY

Trend data provide a dynamic rather than a fixed view of the health status of the MCH population and of the services and systems that can have an impact on that health status. For trend data to be most useful, it is critical that an analysis be conceptually tied to program and policy issues. The job of the analyst, therefore, is to present graphs, tables, statistical results, and narrative that make these connections. In particular, the ability to appropriately analyze and interpret trends for small geographic areas or for small populations is essential if program intervention strategies are to be more targeted and thus more effective.

The scientific literature contains many examples of trend analysis, both theoretical and applied. Attached is a list of articles selected for their relevance to public health practice and in particular for their relevance to maternal and child health. The list is neither comprehensive nor exhaustive, but includes articles that are illustrative of the range of analytic approaches used when examining trend data.

TECHNICAL NOTE ON CONFIDENCE BANDS AND CONFIDENCE LIMITS

A *confidence band* for an estimated regression line is analogous to a confidence interval for a single estimated statistic. With a confidence band, we are measuring the precision of using the regression line to compute the predicted value for an outcome variable (Y) from some particular value of an independent variable (X). For trend analysis, Y may be a rate observed for each calendar year and X may be the values of calendar year, such as 1990, 1991, etc. The standard error of the regression line at any $year_0$ is computed as follows:

$$s.e. = \sqrt{\frac{\sum_{i=1}^{n}(r_i - \hat{r}_i)^2}{n-2}\left(\frac{1}{n} + \frac{(year_0 - \overline{year})}{\sum_{i=1}^{n}(year_i - \overline{year})^2}\right)}$$

where r_i are the observed rates,
$\hat{r}_i$ are the predicted rates (values of the regression line),
n is the number of years being analyzed,
$year_0$ is a particular year,
and $\overline{year}$ is the mean of the year values

Notice how the different components of the formula affect the standard error:

The larger $\sum_{i=1}^{n}(r_i - \hat{r}_i)^2$ (the scatter or variation around the regression line), the larger the standard error predicting the rate at any $year_0$.

The larger the n or sample size (the number of years), the smaller the standard error predicting the rate at any $year_0$.

The larger $\sum_{i=1}^{n}(year_i - \overline{year})^2$ (the variation across the range of years), the smaller the error predicting the rate at any $year_0$.

Finally, the farther away $year_0$ is from $\overline{year}$ (the center of the range of years) the larger the error in predicting the rate.

The 95% confidence interval around each predicted rate is then calculated in the usual manner:

$$\hat{r}_0 \pm 1.96 \sqrt{\frac{\sum\limits_{i=1}^{n}(r_i - \hat{r}_i)^2}{n-2}\left(\frac{1}{n} + \frac{\left(year_0 - \overline{year}\right)}{\sum\limits_{i=1}^{n}\left(year_i - \overline{year}\right)^2}\right)}$$

where $\hat{r}_0$ is the predicted rate at $year_0$

The confidence band around the line is composed of the set of confidence intervals calculated for each data point with the above formula. The band is curved, being narrowest at the center of the observed data and getting progressively wider farther out from the center. In theory, if one were to take repeated samples for the same population and compute the estimated regression line and 95% confidence bands for each sample, then 95% of the computed confidence bands would include the true regression line (in this case, the true trend line) in the population.

When Ordinary Least Squares (OLS) regression is used with trend data, the confidence band as computed above reflects the precision in using a linear equation to predict the rate for any given year, but does not reflect the precision in the rates themselves since the population size giving rise to each observed rate is nowhere accounted for in the formula. In contrast, a confidence interval calculated for a single observed rate addresses the error involved in taking a sample that particular year, but does not incorporate any aspect of changes in rates across different years. Recall the formula for the 95% confidence interval around a rate:

$$r_0 \pm 1.96\sqrt{\frac{r_0}{n}}$$

where n is the number of individuals at risk

Now, population at risk is accounted for, but the formula does not incorporate any of the data from other years, and has no reference to the fitted regression line across years. A 95% confidence interval for a single estimated rate has a 95% chance of including the real rate in the population for that particular year, but connecting a set of these 95% confidence intervals for many years will have less than a 95% chance of including the set of true rates in the population since the 5% error rate in each interval is cumulated across all of the observed rates. A 95% confidence band for the regression line, on the other hand, insures an error rate of 5% for the entire band.

Poisson regression can be used with trend data in an effort to account for both the error in the estimated regression line and the error in the observed data. If the health event of interest is very rare (has a very small probability of occurring), then using logistic regression which models the log-odds of occurrence will be approximately equivalent to using Poisson regression which models the log-rate. The applicability of logistic regression is important because this procedure is more readily available in standard statistical software packages than is Poisson regression. A Poisson or logistic model treats each individual, rather than each year, as an observation with an indicator for whether or not the health event of interest occurred.

Confidence intervals can be computed around the predicted trend line assuming the log-odds of the event changes linearly with time. The logistic regression model for trend data can be written as follows:

$$\ln\left(\frac{p_i}{1-p_i}\right) = \text{intercept} + (\text{slope} \times \text{year}_i)$$

$$\text{where } p_i = \frac{\text{\# of health events in year}_i}{\text{\# in population at risk in year}_i}$$

Once the intercept and slope have been estimated from the data, the predicted probability of the event at year i can be computed. The upper and lower confidence limits for the predicted probability at each year are then computed as a function of the standard errors of the estimates of the intercept and slope. The formula for these standard errors and the confidence band around the set of predicted probabilities from a logistic regression model is beyond the scope of this discussion, except to emphasize that it assesses both the variation around the predicted regression line (as in Ordinary Least Squares regression) and the total at risk across all years.

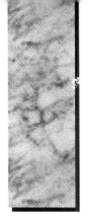

Methods for Analyzing
Trend Data Exercise and Solution

LLBWRATE is the variable name for the natural logarithm of the low birthweight percents.

Area 100 represents the combined data for Chicago Community Areas 33 and 35.
Area 99 represents the data for Chicago as a whole.

The YEAR variable is coded 74, 75, 76, ... , 92, 93, 94.

The values for the parameter estimates are also referred to as the beta coefficients or as the intercept and the slope.

1. Using the SAS® output from modeling the natural log of the low birthweight percents for Chicago community areas 33 and 35 combined, calculate the average annual % change in low birthweight.

Model: MODEL1

 Dependent Variable: LLBWRATE

 Area = 100 (33 & 35 Combined)

 Analysis of Variance

Source	DF	Sum of Squares	Mean Square	F Value	Prob>F
Model	1	0.06504	0.06504	7.760	0.0146
Error	14	0.11733	0.00838		
C Total	15	0.18236			

Root MSE	0.09154	R-square	0.3566	
Dep Mean	2.71827	Adj R-sq	0.3107	
C.V.	3.36777			

Parameter Estimates

Variable	DF	Parameter Estimate	Standard Error	T for H0: Parameter=0	Prob > |T|
INTERCEP	1	1.521931	0.43005775	3.539	0.0033
YEAR	1	0.013831	0.00496472	2.786	0.0146

The results of the regression analysis show that the increase in the low birthweight percent over time in these areas is statistically significant at p = 0.0146. Do you think this is a significant deterioration in low birthweight % from a public health point of view?

2. Using the same output, calculate a projected low birthweight % for the year 2000. Remember that the YEAR variable is coded 79-94.

3. and 4. Using the SAS® output below, repeat questions 1 and 2 for the city of Chicago as a whole.

```
Model: MODEL1

 Dependent Variable: LLBWRATE

 Area = 99 (Chicago)

 Analysis of Variance
```

		Sum of	Mean		
Source	DF	Squares	Square	F Value	Prob>F
Model	1	0.00772	0.00772	20.896	0.0004
Error	14	0.00517	0.00037		
C Total	15	0.01289			

Root MSE	0.01922	R-square	0.5988
Dep Mean	2.35711	Adj R-sq	0.5701
C.V.	0.81525		

```
Parameter Estimates
```

		Parameter	Standard	T for H0:	
Variable	DF	Estimate	Error	Parameter=0	Prob > |T|
INTERCEP	1	1.945033	0.09027388	21.546	0.0001
YEAR	1	0.004764	0.00104215	4.571	0.0004

5. If the city were determined to reach the Year 2000 Objective on time, what would the average annual % decrease in low birthweight have to be given its rate of 10.7 % as of 1994?

6. Community Area 34 is adjacent to Community Areas 33 and 35. Speculate as to the reasons that areas 33 and 35 were combined for analysis, while area 34 was not.

Solutions

1. The average annual % change is low birthweight in areas 33 and 35 combined is:

    $$\left(e^{0.013831} - 1\right) \times 100 = 1.39$$

    This 1.39 % increase per year in low birthweight percent does seem important, especially in light of the decrease in the infant mortality rate over the same time period.

2. The projected low birthweight % in areas 33 and 35 combined in the year 2000 is:

    $$e^{1.521931 + (0.013831 \times 100)} = 18.3$$

    Note that the beta coefficient, or slope, is multiplied by 100 since this is the representation of the year 2000 that follows from the coding of 79-94 for the observed data.

3. The average annual % change is low birthweight in Chicago is:

    $$\left(e^{0.004764} - 1\right) \times 100 = 0.48$$

    Even the 0.48 % increase in low birthweight is a signal that progress is not being made in improving the health status of newborns in the city. The p-value is highly significant because of the stability, and therefore, the smoothness in the yearly low birthweight percents.

4. The projected low birthweight % in Chicago in the year 2000 is:

    $$e^{1.945033 + (0.004764 \times 100)} = 11.3$$

    Again, 100 is used to represent the year 2000.

5. In order for the city to reach a low birthweight % of 5, given the 1994 rate of 10.7%, the average annual percent decrease would have to be:

    $$\left(\frac{\frac{5 - 10.7}{10.7}}{6} \right) \times 100 = -8.9$$

    Reducing the low birthweight percent by 8.9% per year would be very dramatic, and very difficult to achieve.

6. Areas 33 and 35 are quite similar (homogeneous) on demographic as well as health status measures. In order to increase sample size, and thus the stability of rates, the data for these two similar areas are combined. Area 34, though close geographically, is somewhat different than the other two areas on important factors, and combining its data with the data for the other two areas might obscure these differences. In addition to demographic homogeneity and the desire to increase sample size, service delivery issues and planning of intervention strategies may guide whether areas are considered jointly or separately.

Selected Bibliography

1. Alexander, J.A., M.T. Halperin, and S.Y. Lee. 1996. The short-term effects of merger on hospital operations. Health Services Research. 30: 827-847.

2. Bailey, N.T.J. 1994. Estimating HIV incidence and AIDS Projections: prediction and validation in the public health modeling of HIV/AIDS. *Statistics in Medicine*. 13: 1933-1943.

3. Becker, S.R., F. Diop, and J.N. Thornton. 1993. Infant and child mortality in two counties of Liberia: Results of a survey in 1988 and trends since 1984. *Int. J. Epidemiol*. 22: S56-S63.

4. Bhat, P.N., K. Navaneetham, and S.I. Rajan. 1995. Maternal mortality in India: estimates from a regression model. Stud. Fam. Plann. 26: 217-232.

5. Boyle, P. and C. Robertson. 1987. Statistical modeling of lung cancer and laryngeal cancer incidence in Scotland, 1960-1979. *Amer. J. Epidemiol*. 125: 731-744.

6. Breslow, N.E. 1984. Extra-Poisson variation in log-linear models. *Appl. Statist*. 33:38-44.

7. Brillinger, D.R. 1986. A biometrics invited paper with discussion: the natural variability of vital rates and associated statistics. *Biometrics* 42: 693-734.

8. Brookmeyer, R. and M.H. Gail. 1988. A method for obtaining short-term projections and lower bounds on the size of the AIDS epidemic. *J. Amer. Statist. Assoc*. 83: 301-308.

9. Buescher, P.A. 1996. Smoking in pregnancy in North Carolina: maternal characteristics and trends 1988-1994. State Center for Health Statistics No. 101.

10. Catalano, R. and S. Serxner. 1987. Time series designs of potential interest to epidemiologists. *Amer. J. Epidemiol*. 126: 724-731.

11. Chaulk, C.P., K. Moore-Rice, R. Rizzo, and R.R. Chaisson. 1995. Eleven years of community-based directly observed therapy for tuberculosis. *JAMA* 274: 945-951.

12. Chin, J. and S.K. Lwanga. 1991. Estimation and projection of adult AIDS cases: a simple epidemiological model. WHO Bulletin OMS 69: 399-406.

13. Davis, H., K.C. Schoendorf, P.J. Gergen and R.M. Moore. 1997. National trends in the mortality of children with Sickle Cell Disease, 1968 through 1992. *Amer. J. Public Health* 87:1317-1322.

14. Devesa, S.S., J Donaldson, and T. Fears. 1995. Graphical presentation of trends in rates. *Amer. J. Epidemiol*. 141: 300-304.

15. Downs, A.M., R.A. Ancelle-Park, and J.B. Brunet. 1990. Surveillance of AIDS in the European community: recent trends and predictions to 1991. AIDS 4: 1117-1124.

16. Geddes, J.R. and E. Juszczak. 1995. Period trends in rate of suicide in first 28 days after discharge from psychiatric hospital in Scotland, 1968-1992. BMJ 311: 357-360.

17. Glynn, R.J., T.A. Stukel, S.M. Sharp, T.A. Bubolz, J.L. Freeman, and E.S. Fisher. 1993. Estimating the variance of standardized rates of recurrent events, with application to hospitalizations among the elderly in New England. *Amer. J. Epidemiol.* 137: 776-786.

18. Greenland, S. 1995. Dose-response and trend analysis in Epidemiology: alternatives to categorical analysis. *Epidemiol* 6: 356-365.

19. Hakulinen, T. and T. Dyba. 1994. Precision of incidence predictions based on Poisson distributed observations. *Statist. In Med.* 13: 1513-1523.

20. Hamers, F.F., T.A. Peterman, A.A. Zaida, R.L. Ranson, J.E. Wrotten, and J.J. Witte. 1995. Syphilis and gonorrhea in Miami: similar clustering, different trends. *Amer. J. Public Health* 85: 1104-1108.

21. Helfenstein, U. 1991. The use of transfer function models, intervention analysis and related time series methods in epidemiology. *Intern. J. Epidemiol.* 20: 808-815.

22. Hodge, M.J., G.E. Dougherty, I.B. Pless. 1995. Pediatric mortality and hospital use in Canada and the United States, 1971 through 1987. *Amer. J. Public Health* 85: 1276-1279.

23. Janerich, D.T. 1984. Forecasting cancer trends to optimize control strategies. *JNCI* 72: 1317-1321.

24. Katzenellenbogen, J., D. Yach, and R.E. Dorrington. 1993. Mortality in a rural South African mission, 1837-1909: an historical cohort study using church records. Intern, J. Epidemiol. 22: 965-973.

25. Keiding, N., P.K. Anderson, and K. Frederiksen. 1990. Modeling excess mortality of the unemployed: choice of scale and extra-Poisson variability. *Appl. Stats.* 39: 63-74.

26. Kleinman, J. 1991. Methodological issues in the analysis of vital statistics. In *Reproductive and Perinatal Epidemiology*, Kiely, M. ed., Boston: CRC press.

27. Kuhn, L., L.L. Davidson, and M.S. Durkin. 1994. Use of Poisson regression and time series analysis for detecting changes over time in rates of child injury following a prevention program. *Amer. J. Epidemiol.* 140: 943 – 955.

28. Land, G.H. and J.W. Stockbauer. 1993. Smoking and pregnancy outcome: trends among black teenage mothers in Missouri. *Amer. J. Public Health.* 83: 1121-1124.

29. MacNeill, I.B., J.M. Elwood, D. Miller, and Y. Mao. 1995. Trends in mortality from melanoma in Canada and prediction of future rates. *Stat. Med.* 14: 821-839.

30. Malcolm, M.S. and C.E. Salmond. 1993. Trends in amenable mortality in New Zealand 1968-1987. *Intern. J. Epidemiol.* 22: 468-474.

31. Morbidity and Mortality Weekly Report. 1994. Surveillance for selected tobacco-use behaviors – United States, 1900-1994. CDC Surveillance Summaries Vol. 43, No. SS-3.

32. Morbidity and Mortality Weekly Report. 1995. Trends in smoking initiation among adolescents and young adults--United Stated, 1980-1989. 44: 521-525.

33. Morbidity and Mortality Weekly Report. 1995. Pertussis—United States, January, 1992-June, 1995. 44: 525-529.

34. Morbidity and Mortality Weekly Report. 1995. Pneumonia and influenza death rates– United States, 1979-1994. 44: 535-537.

35. Morbidity and Mortality Weekly Report. 1995. State-specific changes in physical activity among persons aged 65 or older—United States, 1987-1992. 44: 669-673.

36. Murray, D.M. 1995. Design and analysis of community trials: lessons from the Minnesota heart health program. *Amer. J. Epidemiol.* 142: 569-575.

37. Nam. J.M. 1995. Interval estimation and significance testing for cyclic trends in seasonality studies. *Biometrics* 51: 1411-1417.

38. Nelson, D.E., G.A. Giovino, D.R. Shopland, P.D. Mowery, S.L. Mills, and M.P. Eriksen. 1995. Trends in cigarette smoking among US adolescents, 1974 through 1991. *Amer. J. Public Health.* 85:34-40.

39. Opitz, W. and H. Nelson. 1996. Short-term, population-based forecasting in the public sector. *Popul. Res. Policy Rev.* 15:549-563.

40. Parker, R.A. 1989. Analysis of surveillance data with Poisson regression: a case study. *Statist. In Med.* 8: 285-294.

41. Polednak, A.P. 1994. Projected numbers of cancers diagnosed in the US elderly population, 1990-2030. *Amer. J. Public Health* 84: 1313-1316.

42. Rockett, I.R.H. and J.H. Pollard. 1995. Life table analysis of the United States' year 2000 mortality objectives. *Intern. J. Epidemiol.* 24: 547-551.

43. Ruwaar, D., R.T. Hoogenveen, H. Verkleif, D. Kromhout, A.F. Casparie, and E. A. van der Veen. 1993. Forecasting the number of diabetic patients in the Netherlands in 2005. *Amer. J. Public Health* 83: 989-995.

44. Sankrithi, U, I. Emanuel, and G. van Belle. 1991. Comparison of linear and exponential multivariate models for explaining national infant and child mortality. *Intern. J. Epidemiol* 20: 565-570.

45. Singh, G.K., and S.M. Yu. 1995. Infant mortality in the United States: trends, differentials, and projections, 1950-2010. *Amer. J. Public Health* 85:957-964.

46. Siskind, V., C. Del Mar, and F. Schofield. 1993. Infant feeding in Queensland, Australia: long-term trends. *Amer. J. Public Health.* 83: 103-106.

47. Thomas, J.C., A.L. Kulik and V.J. Schoenbach. 1995. Syphilis in the south: rural rates surpass urban rates in North Carolina. *Amer. J. Public Health* 85:1119-1122.

48. Tuomilehto, J., E. Virtala, M. Karvonen, R. Lounamaa, J. Pitkamiemi, R. Reunanen, E. Tuomilehto-Wolf, L. Toivanen, and the Dime Study Group. 1995. Increase in incidence of insulin-dependent diabetes mellitus among children in Finland. *Intern. J. Public Health* 24: 984-992.

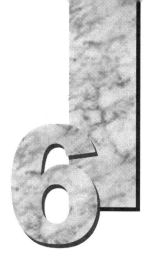

Creating Target Population Estimates Using National Survey Data

by Colleen Monahan, DC, MPH

Maternal and child health (MCH) programs target a wide variety of population groups for services. One targeted group, in particular, is children with special health care needs (CSHCN). Estimating the size of the population, including relevant subgroups is a core function of MCH/CSHCN programs.

This module was developed to assist state and local program staff in developing these estimates for this group.

This module will address:

- Describing target population characteristics
- Sources of data
- Developing indirect estimates of a target population
- Developing a state synthetic population estimate
- Exercises and Solutions
- References

DESCRIBING TARGET POPULATION CHARACTERISTICS FOR CHILDREN WITH SPECIAL HEALTH CARE NEEDS

Illuminating the characteristics of the population of interest is the first step toward estimating the size of the target population. Target populations may be defined by age and sex (e.g., teen family planning, adolescent health, etc.), program eligibility (e.g., children with special health care needs, SSI, school health clinics, Ryan White Fund, etc.) or income level (e.g., Healthy Start, Medicaid, etc.). Populations defined by race, age, sex or income can often be directly estimated using census data.

When population characteristics cannot be measured using Census data, topical sample surveys are the next best source of data. However, because we often do not have this type of locally collected data, more complex estimation procedures are required such as synthetic estimation. (Refer to Module 3 for more detailed discussion of synthetic estimation.)

Estimating the population of children with special health care needs has been the biggest challenge for MCH programs. This population was chosen for the focus of this module because it exemplifies many of the issues we face in target population estimation.

WHO ARE CHILDREN WITH SPECIAL HEALTH CARE NEEDS?

Children with special health care needs (CSHCN) include children with a wide variety of health conditions. Some of these children also have more than one condition. Estimation of the number of CSHCN may involve identifying:

- the prevalence of children with special needs as identified by state and federal programs,
- the prevalence of specific diseases and conditions in children,
- the prevalence of functional limitations among children,
- the proportion of children who require or need specialized services, and
- the proportion of children who are regarded by others as disabled.

Because *there is no data source from which a direct measurement of the size of this population* can be estimated and because of the diversity of definitions, no one method alone will completely provide an all-inclusive estimate of the prevalence of CSHCN. Therefore, averaging and/or summing multiple types of estimates may be required. Before we can create an estimate it is important to understand the variety of ways that this population may be defined.

The definition chosen can have major implications for the size of the population estimate as reflected in the following examples (McManus 1997):

- 31% of children have chronic physical conditions
  (1988 Child Health Supplement to National Health Interview Survey)

- 20% of children have chronic mental conditions
  (1988 Child Health Supplement to National Health Interview Survey)

- 7% of children have a limitation of activity
  (1994 Child Health Supplement to National Health Interview Survey)

- 2% of children have a limitation in activities of daily living
  (1978-1980 National Health Interview Survey)

There are three major approaches to defining CSHCN:

- Diagnosis-based,
- Function-based, and
- Service-based.

Diagnosis-Based Approach

There have been widely differing estimates published on children with chronic illness/disability. Because there is no consensus from the research community on a definition, there is an emphasis on reporting single disease/condition prevalence or incidence. Newacheck and Taylor (1992) reported that published estimates range from 5% to more than 30%. They also reported that two or more conditions coexist in about 30% of affected children. In addition, undiagnosed conditions are not counted. Research has shown that there are commonalties in the experience of having a chronic condition, in addition to those specific to a particular condition. However, by focusing in on reporting the prevalence of conditions, the overall experience of the child and family is missed. In addition, when reporting the prevalence of conditions, it is important to distinguish between conditions that are acute, transient and/or self-limited from those which are lengthy in duration or more likely to be permanent. Therefore, knowledge about the length of time that the child has had the condition is critical to developing a prevalence measure which is meaningful to program planning for CSHCN.

Function-Based Approach

Unlike diagnosis, limitations in function have a direct impact on the quality of life and use of resources by CSHCN. Therefore, estimating the prevalence of children with functional limitations can be more useful for program planning than diagnosis. Function may be categorized into four areas: mobility, self-care, communication and learning ability. Self-care and mobility impairments have been associated with lower rates of survivorship (Eyman, et al, 1990) and are the least prevalent among functional limitations in children. The most common functional limitations among children involve communication and learning ability.

Unlike diagnosis, the measurement of limitation is not available in the medical record and actual performance-based measurement is not available in most cases. National population estimates of functional limitation are obtained using standardized questionnaires. Two major surveys which collect this information for persons of all ages include the Survey on Income and Program Participation (SIPP) (http://www.census.gov/hhes/sippdesc.html) conducted by the U.S. Bureau of the Census and the National Health Interview Survey conducted by the National Center for Health Statistics (NCHS). Survey methods for measuring functional limitations are difficult to design due to the age-relatedness of functional limitations.

The major focus of SIPP is on income and the labor force. SIPP concentrates on children ages 6-14 and treats children ages 15-17 as adults. SIPP asks about: ability to perform activities of daily living (ADL's); the use of wheelchairs, canes, crutches and walkers; the ability to perform the functional activities of seeing, hearing, walking, running and using stairs; the ability to do regular schoolwork, and presence of a learning disability, mental retardation or some other developmental disability.

The National Health Interview Survey conducted a special survey on disability in 1994-95 (heretofore called NHIS-D). The NHIS-D included separate questions for children under age 4 and questions very similar to SIPP for children ages 5-17. Measures for functional limitation used in these surveys were developed for various purposes; therefore, there is no single unified approach to estimating the number of children with activity limitations. It is estimated that 2 percent of all disabled children are missed by household-based surveys like NHIS-D (Hogan, et al, 1997), which is much less than the adult disabled because so few children are institutionalized. The NHIS-D showed that 1.3 percent of children have a mobility impairment, 0.9 percent have a self-care impairment, 5.5 percent have a communication limitation and 10.6 percent are limited in their learning ability (Hogan, et al 1997).

While measuring functional limitations has advantages over the diagnosis-based approach, it still has limitations. Using this method by itself may miss children who are functioning well but still need ongoing services or care.

Service-Based Approach

Many CSHCN have a need for specialized services or primary and preventive services at a level above and beyond the level usually needed by children. Estimates developed using this approach would be possible when programs have sufficient service billing information to identify CSHCN. This approach, however, excludes children with chronic conditions who use services in small quantities.

CLASSIFICATION SYSTEMS FOR DISABILITY

How narrowly or broadly one defines the CSHCN population has an impact on estimating a target population. Researchers conducting studies on disability, often use classical frameworks to define the various domains of disability. This is required if a researcher intends to identify persons with different types of disabilities or examine the effect of interventions on the extent of disability. There are three major classification systems used for this purpose: the National Advisory Board on Medical Rehabilitation Research model, the International Classification of Impairments, Disabilities and Handicaps developed by the World Health Organization; and a model proposed by Saad Nagi, from the Institute of Medicine.

The National Advisory Board on Medical Rehabilitation Research Model

The National Advisory Board on Medical Rehabilitation Research, of the National Center for Medical Rehabilitation Research (NCMRR), established within the National Institute for Child Health and Development, developed a disability model following the July 1990 adoption of the Americans with Disabilities Act. The NCMRR model (NIH 1993) presents five aspects of disability:

1. **Pathophysiology:** the interruption of or interference with normal physiological and developmental processes or structures.
2. **Impairment:** the loss or abnormality of cognitive, emotional, physiological, or anatomical structure or function, including all losses or abnormalities, not just those attributable to the initial pathophysiology.
3. **Functional Limitation:** the restriction or lack of ability to perform an action in the manner or with the range consistent with the purpose of an organ or organ system.
4. **Disability:** the inability or limitation in performing tasks, activities, and roles to levels expected in physical and social contexts.
5. **Societal Limitation:** the restriction, attributable to social policy or barriers (structural and attitudinal), which limits fulfillment of roles or denies access to services and opportunities that are associated with full participation in society.

International Classification of Impairments, Disabilities, and Handicaps (ICIDH)

The ICIDH model presents four aspects of disability:

1. **Disease:** the presence of a diagnosed condition.
2. **Impairment:** any loss or abnormality of psychological, physiological, or anatomical structure or function.
3. **Disability:** a restriction in the ability to perform essential components of everyday living.
4. **Handicap:** a limitation on the fulfillment of a role that is normal for that individual.

According to ICIDH a "handicap" is a consequence of a "disability" and a "disability" is a consequence of an "impairment." However, impairments do not necessarily lead to disabilities, nor do disabilities necessarily lead to handicaps. Most importantly, this model suggests a detailed classification system that offers the potential for detailed needs assessment.

Institute of Medicine/Saad Nagi Model

The NCMRR model builds heavily on the Nagi model. The Nagi model presents four aspects of disability:

1. **Pathology:** interruption or interference of normal bodily processes (at the cellular level).
2. **Impairment:** any loss or abnormality of psychological, physiological, or anatomical structure or function.
3. **Functional Limitation:** restriction or lack of ability to perform an action or activity in a manner considered normal that results from an impairment.
4. **Disability:** a restriction in the ability to perform essential components of everyday living.

OTHER MODELS OR DEFINITIONS OF DISABILITY

Framework Proposed by Ruth Stein, et al, for the QuiCCC

Ruth Stein, et al (1993) developed a questionnaire for identifying children with chronic conditions (QuiCCC) based on a conceptual framework also developed by her and her colleagues.

This framework defines ongoing health conditions as disorders that:

   I. Have a biologic, psychologic, or cognitive basis, and
  II. Have lasted or are virtually certain to last for at least 1 year, and
III. Produce one or more of the following sequelae:
     A. Limitation of function, activities, or social role in comparison with age peers in the general areas of physical, cognitive, emotional, and social growth and development.
     B. Dependency on one of the following to compensate for or minimize limitation of function, activities, or social role:
         1. Medications
         2. Special diet
         3. Medical technology

4. Assistive device
5. Personal assistance

C. Need for medical care or related services, psychological services or educational services over and above the usual for the child's age, or for special ongoing treatments, interventions, or accommodations at home or in school.

National Association of Children's Hospitals and Related Institutions (NACHRI) Classification System

The National Association of Children's Hospitals and Related Institutions (NACHRI) developed a classification system to identify individuals who have a congenital or chronic condition expected to last 12 months or longer (Muldoon, et al 1997). The system relies on the International Classification of Diseases, Ninth Edition, Clinical Modification (ICD-9-CM) codes that classify chronic disease by body system, condition category, severity level and disease progression. Acute conditions are not included in this system.

The following are key concepts of the NACHRI system:

Chronic health condition: defined as a physical, mental, emotional, behavioral or developmental disorder expected to last 12 months or longer or having sequelae that last 12 months or longer and requires treatment or monitoring. Approximately 4,000 of the 15,000 ICD-9-CM codes met these criteria.
Severity level of diagnosis: each diagnosis is given an initial severity level based on expected complexities and costliness of all health care services over a 12-month period.
Severity level of person: each person is assigned a severity level based on the severity level of the diagnosis, disease progression, interactive effects of multiple conditions, and supplemental status indicators.
Disease progression: each diagnosis is assigned to a disease progression type based on the expected course of the disease and treatment goal: cure/substantially improve, substantially improve/continuous treatment, status/improve function, progressive, supportive care, or mixed course.
"At-risk" categories: conditions that do not meet the criteria used for a chronic condition but usually require services of an amount and type greater than that for not chronically ill persons and place the individual at risk for a chronic condition.

The NACHRI approach is limited in that it relies on the accuracy of the ICD-9-CM codes and on the medical diagnosis. Its use involves the analysis of very large claims data sets, such as Medicaid and hospital claims data.

Definition from the Federal Bureau of Maternal and Child Health

The federal Bureau of Maternal and Child Health (of the Health Resources and Services Administration (HRSA) in the Department of Health and Human Services (DHHS) which administers the Title V MCH Block Grant) defines children with special health care needs as:

"...those children who have or are at increased risk for chronic physical, developmental, behavioral, or emotional conditions and who require health and related services of a type or amount beyond that required by children generally."

The definition includes the following types of children: children with a diagnosis of a chronic illness, children who require services, and children at-risk. State Children with Special Health Care Needs programs (funded under Title V) have historically targeted cardiovascular, neurological and orthopedic conditions such as congenital heart defects, cerebral palsy and spina bifida. These types of conditions have a relatively stable incidence and prevalence and are relatively rare and therefore can be estimated reliably. However, there are a group of conditions that are new and/or increasing or changing in prevalence and incidence. These conditions include psychiatric, emotional and learning disorders, chronic infectious diseases (e.g., AIDS, hepatitis, etc.) and asthma.

Definition Using State Program Eligibility

The target population of CSHCN may be described using program *diagnostic eligibility*. This definition usually includes diagnostic, age and income criteria. Although this definition is limited to those eligible for a program, it can be useful to focus on a population that the program is in a position to address or a population that is "convenient" to measure. Program definitions that may be used include SSI, rehabilitation services and special education. It may also be helpful to compare the size of the population served by each program and how that population is geographically distributed within a state.

Americans with Disabilities Act (ADA)

The Americans with Disabilities Act (ADA) defines an individual as having a disability if the individual meets one of the following criteria:

1. have a physical or mental impairment that limits one or more of the major life activities,
2. have a record of such impairment, or
3. be regarded as having such an impairment.

This definition is important in that many legal battles over access for the "disabled" will be fought based on it. Any person attempting to access any public service or structure, who requests assistance or reduction in physical barriers due to having a disability, will be judged according to this definition.

The Physical-Mental Continuum

The Research Consortium on Chronic Illness in Childhood has identified a Physical-Mental continuum for describing a child with a chronic health condition. Each item on the continuum has a low and high end of a scale identified.

Duration	Brief----------------------------	Lengthy
Age of onset	Congenital----------------------	Acquired
Limitation of age-appropriate activities	None----------------------------	Unable to conduct
Visibility	Not visible----------------------	Highly visible
Expected survival	Usual longevity----------------	Immediate threat to life
Mobility	Not impaired------------------	Extremely impaired
Physiologic functioning	Not impaired------------------	Extremely impaired
Cognition	Normal------------------------	Extremely impaired
Emotional/social	Normal------------------------	Extremely impaired
Sensory functioning	Not impaired------------------	Extremely impaired
Communication	Not impaired------------------	Extremely impaired
Course	Stable--------------------------	Progressive
Uncertainty	Episodic------------------------	Predictable

THE ROLE OF SOCIODEMOGRAPHIC FACTORS IN ESTIMATING DISABILITY

Socioeconomic status is a fundamental correlate of disease because it affects access to important resources as well as affects whether an individual is exposed to harmful agents or hazards (Hogan, et al, 1997). The sociodemographic circumstances of a child's family circumstances are central to the understanding of disability, including identification, diagnosis, treatment and rehabilitation response (Newacheck 1992). Sociodemographic characteristics should always be examined when estimating children with disability. These characteristics include race and ethnicity, household structure (number of parents in household, other adults), education of guardians and family income (or presence of poverty).

SOURCES OF DATA ON DISABILITY

The Census Bureau

The Census Bureau (http://www.census.gov) collects a significant amount of information on disability status. The long form questionnaire on the 1990 Decennial census contained questions about disability, including questions about work disability, the ability to go outside the home alone, and the ability to take care of personal needs. This data set is the only one that can provide direct estimates of disability at sub-state geographic levels. Following the 1990 census, a Content Reinterview Survey was conducted which provided more specific information on limitations. Although the majority of the disability information is on the adult population, adult disability status can be used to establish need for and use of community resources. For example, if the unemployment status is higher for persons with disability in one community compared with another, it can be argued that increased resources should be applied to CSHCN in preparing them for transition to adulthood (e.g., job training, education, etc.).

The Census Bureau conducts three major surveys: the Decennial Census, Survey on Income and Program Participation, and the Current Population Survey (see *Module 7*).

The Survey on Income and Program Participation (SIPP)
The SIPP (http://www.census.gov/hhes/sippdesc.html) is a national household survey that began in 1984. An extensive and reasonably consistent set of questions relating to disability was asked in 1990, 1991, 1992 and 1993 SIPP. This survey is the preferred source among Census Bureau surveys for disability information. The disadvantage to using these data is the small sample size that restricts the use of the data below the regional level.

The Current Population Survey
The Current Population Survey (CPS) (http://www.bls.census.gov/cps/cpsmain.htm) is conducted monthly and the disability questions focus only on work. The CPS identifies persons who are out of the labor force because of a disability and, in each March survey since 1980, identifies persons who have health problems which "prevent them from working or limits the kind or amount of work they can do."

The National Center for Health Statistics

 The National Center for Health Statistics (NCHS) of the U.S. Department of Health and Human Services (DHHS) is the primary Federal source of data on the physical health of the U.S. population. The NCHS collects and publishes data on a variety of health topics.

The National Health Interview Survey

The National Health Interview Survey (NHIS) (http://www.cdc.gov/nchswww/index.htm) is one of the major surveys of the National Center for Health Statistics (NCHS), Centers for Disease Control and Prevention (http://www.cdc.gov/). Through NHIS, information concerning the health of the civilian noninstitutionalized population is collected through household interviews conducted throughout the United States. Each year, the survey consists of a basic set of questions on health, socioeconomic, and demographic items as well as one or more special questionnaires to obtain more detailed information on major current health issues. The NHIS has operated continuously since 1957, and its sample survey design has been reevaluated and modified following each of the last three decennial censuses of the U.S. population.

The core questionnaire includes the following types of basic health and demographic questions:

1. Demographic characteristics of household members, including age, sex, race, education, and family income.
2. Disability days, including restricted-activity and bed disability days, and work- and school-loss days occurring during the 2-week period prior to the week of interview, as well as days spent in bed during the last 12 months.
3. Physician visits occurring during the same 2-week period, the interval since the last physician visit, and the number of visits during the last 12 months.
4. Acute and chronic conditions responsible for these days and visits.
5. Long-term limitation of activity resulting from chronic disease or impairment and the chronic conditions associated with the disability.
6. Short-stay hospitalization data, including the number of hospital episodes during the past year and the number of days for each stay.

Interviews are conducted each week throughout the year in a probability sample of households. The interviewing is performed by a permanent staff of interviewers employed by the U.S. Bureau of the Census. Data collected over the period of a year form the basis for the development of annual estimates of the health characteristics of the population and for the analysis of trends in those characteristics.
All adult members of the household 17 years of age and older who are at home at the time of the interview are invited to participate and to respond for themselves. Information for children and for adults not at home during the interview is provided by a responsible adult (19 years of age and over) residing in the household. Between 65 and 70 percent of the adults 17 years of age and over are self-respondents. Generally, a random subsample of adult household members is selected to self-respond to additional questions on current health topics that vary from year to year. Depending on the household size and the nature and extent of health conditions of household members, the length of the interview ranges between 20 and 90 minutes.

The households selected for interview each week are a probability sample representative of the target population. Data are collected from approximately 49,000 households including about 132,000 persons in a calendar year. Participation is voluntary; confidentiality of responses is guaranteed. The annual response rate of NHIS is over 95 percent of the eligible households in the sample.

National Health Interview Survey Supplements Relevant to Children's Health

NHIS 1990 Special Topics:
- Assistive Devices

NHIS 1991 Special Topics:
- Unintentional injuries

- Child health (includes childhood immunization; use of seat belts and safety seats; use of headgear and mouth guards during organized athletic activities; and, information on functional disabilities)
- Health promotion and disease prevention

NHIS 1992 Special Topics:
- Youth Risk Behavior Survey (youths 12-24)

NHIS 1993 Special Topics:
- Childhood immunizations (children <6 in each family with age-eligible children)
- Family resources (asked about all family members)

NHIS 1994 Special Topic:
- Survey on Disability (see below)

National Health Interview Survey on Disability
The National Disability Survey
(http://www.cdc.gov/nchswww/products/catalogs/subject/nhis/diswrit.htm) is the first comprehensive survey of persons with disabilities, including children with disabilities. The survey was administered in two separate phases in 1994-95. Phase I included core NHIS items and a special set of items related to disability. This survey was intended to serve as a screen to identify persons with disabilities. Phase II was administered 6 to 9 months after Phase I to persons identified in Phase I as having a disability. The phase I survey was administered to 73,000 households with a total of 186,000 individuals.

Proposed data release dates are as follows:

Phase 1, 1994: July 1996
Phase 1, 1995: January 1998
Phase 2, 1994: February 1998
Phase 2, 1995: March 1998

Other Relevant Surveys Conducted by NCHS
National Hospital Discharge Survey (NHDS)
The NHDS (http://www.cdc.gov/nchswww/products/catalogs/subject/nhds/nhds.htm) is a continuing na-tionwide sample survey that gathers information each year on patients (excluding newborn infants) dis-charged from a sample of non-Federal short-stay and specialty hospitals in the U.S. Unfortunately, be-cause relatively few children are hospitalized each year and the NHDS does not oversample the child population, estimates are unreliable except for the most prevalent conditions.

Longitudinal Follow-up to the National Maternal and Infant Health Survey (1991)
This survey (http://www.cdc.gov/nchswww/products/catalogs/subject/mihs/lfnmihs.htm) was conducted among mothers who were initially identified in the 1988 National Maternal and Infant Health Survey (NMIHS). Information contained on this survey may be linked to the birth outcomes identified in the NMIHS survey. Extensive information was obtained about the mother and child, making this survey one of the most important resources for health information on children ages 3 to 4 years of age.

USING NATIONAL DATA TO DEVELOP SYNTHETIC ESTIMATES

National surveys are conducted using sampling methods that provide reliable and valid estimates for the United States as a whole and for very large subregions (e.g., West, South, etc.). Sample size and sampling design prevent the use of these data to provide direct estimates for smaller geographic areas. In order to make state and local estimates of measures from national surveys, synthetic estimates may be used. This involves applying summary proportions generated from the national data and applying them to state or local census data.

Synthetic estimation involves the use of values of a variable of interest from a geographic area and/or time period other than the geographic area and time period of the estimate being produced.

Before discussing synthetic estimation further, other considerations of using national survey data must be understood.

National Survey Data Are Weighted
In a national sample survey, such as the National Health Interview Survey, each individual is assigned a weight based on a complex sampling design. Some groups are oversampled. When analyzing weighted data, analysis must account for each individual's weight. After weighting is accounted for, the final estimate represents the total number of individuals for the nation. For example, a sample of 16,000 persons may represent, in the analysis, 24 million persons. Information about how the data were weighted is usually available in the documentation which accompanies the file. In the NHIS data files each record includes a variable which accounts for that individual's total weight in the survey.

Using Published Tables to Obtain Indirect Estimates
In lieu of using a data file to develop estimates, one can use published data tables. Advantages of using published tables are that the estimates are already weighted and that no data processing skills are required. The primary disadvantage to this method is that you must use the estimates and the stratification groups provided by the authors.

Creating Estimates from a Data File Directly
Using the data file itself offers more flexibility to create a greater number of estimates for a variety of population groups. The majority of national survey data are now available in CD format and packaged with software to allow some manipulation of the data file.

Creating a Synthetic Estimate

All of the national data-sets discussed above can be used to create synthetic estimates of the target population of CSHCN. The following example shows how a synthetic estimate can be calculated for the number of children ages 17 years and under with activity limitation in State X. The formula below shows the weighted percent of children with activity limitation to be 6.8 percent (taken from the 1994 NHIS Disability Supplement) using the data from the table on the next page.

$$\frac{4,743,842}{70,023,660} = 0.068$$

Characteristic	All ages 17 years and under
All children	70,023,660
Activity Status	
Not limited	65,279,818 (93.2%)
Limited	4,743,842 (6.8%)

If the number of children ages 0-17 in State X is 800,000 then the estimated number of children with activity limitation in State X is 53,600. This was obtained using the following formula:

proportion of children with activity $\times$ the number of children $=$ the estimate of the number
limitations in the national survey   in State X   of children with activity
                                                    limitations in State X
                                                         or
                                           using actual numbers:
                               $0.0068 \times 800,000 = 54,400$

In many cases these synthetic estimates are better than the direct estimate collected locally. This is because many local data collection efforts fail to have adequate sample size to generate stable estimates for many populations of interest.

Potential Biases Associated with Creating Synthetic Estimates

Using data that have not been collected directly from the population of interest can introduce potential bias in the estimates that one should be aware of. Biases may differ depending on the application because the synthetic estimate will be a better representation of reality in some population domains than in others. To use national data to estimate target populations in ALL areas, the data must be stratified on population characteristics related to the indicator being estimated (e.g., age, sex, etc.).

Developing a State Estimate for CSHCN

The first step in developing an estimate is to identify which characteristics of CSHCN you want to measure. Refer to the discussion on defining the population in Module 1 and refer to the section on synthetic estimates in Module 3 for more information on the method. Tables 1-8 may be found on pages 249-254.

Tables used in the exercises were produced using the *SETS* software that accompanies the CD-ROM version of the 1994 National Health Interview Survey on Disability (NHIS-DS). All estimates are based on weighted data. The state data table was created using data from the Census Bureau, also available on CD-ROM.

Table 3 includes age stratified estimates of children with activity limitation (taken from the NHIS-DS). Table 2 includes summary data by age and poverty status for State X.

What is the expected number of children in State X ages 0-5 with activity limitation?

Table 3 shows the stratified estimate of children ages 0 to 5 with activity limitation to be 830,996 or 3.4% of children surveyed in the age group.
Table 2 shows the number of children ages 0 to 5 in State X to be 1,018,444.

The synthetic estimate of children ages 0 to 5 years with activity limitation can be computed as:

$$1,018,444 \times 0.034 = 34,627 \text{ children}$$

What is the expected number of children in State X ages 0-11 with activity limitation?

Table 3 shows the stratified estimate of children with activity limitation from the national data-set:

ages 0 to 5	3.4%
ages 6 to 11	8.3%

Table 2 shows the following number of children in these age strata in State X:

ages 0 to 5	1,018,444
ages 6 to 11	1,211,253

The synthetic estimate of children ages 0 to 11 years with activity limitation can be computed as:

Age	National Estimate	State X Population	Synthetic Estimate
ages 0 to 5	3.4%	1,018,444	34,627
ages 6 to 11	8.3%	1,211,253	100,534
Total		2,229,697	135,161

135,161 / 2,229,697 = 0.061 or 6.1%

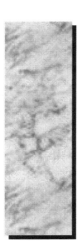

Creating Target Population Estimates Using National Survey Data
Exercises and Solutions

The data used in this exercise section are from the National Health Interview Survey on Disability, Phase 1, developed by the National Center for Health Statistics (NCHS). Tables 1, and 3 through 8 provide the data on some characteristics of the children with special health care needs (CSHCN). These tables were produced using the *SETS* software that accompanies the CD-ROM version of the 1994 National Health Interview Survey on Disability. Table 2 includes summary data by age and poverty status for State X. These type of data are also available on CD format from the Census Bureau on Summary Tape File 3.

Exercise 1
Estimating the number of children with a specified condition

Table 1 provides a sample of prevalence measures.
Table 2 contains summary population data for State X.

Use information from Table 1 and Table 2 to answer the following questions:

a.   What is the expected number of children ages 0-5 in State X with a learning disability?
b.   What is the expected number of children ages 0-17 in State X with cerebral palsy?

Exercise 2
Estimating the number of children with diminished functional status

Table 3 provides a sample of proportions of children with functional limitations.
Table 2 contains summary population data for State X.

Use information from Table 2 and Table 3 to answer the following questions:

a.   What is the expected number of children in State X ages 12-17 having difficulty with strenuous activity?

b. What is the expected number of children in State X ages 0-17 with activity limitation?

Exercise 3
Estimating the number of children with a need for specialized services

Table 4 provides a sample of summary data describing health service utilization among children. Table 2 contains summary population data for State X.

Use information from Table 2 and Table 4 to answer the following questions:

a. What is the expected number of children in State X ages 12-17 who visit a doctor or specialist on a regular basis?
b. What is the expected number of children in State X ages 0-17 who receive therapy in or out of the home?

Exercise 4
Estimating the number of children considered by others to have a disability

Table 5 provides sample proportions of children considered by others to have a disability. Table 2 contains summary population data for State X.

Use information from Table 2 and Table 5 to answer the following questions:

a. What is the expected number of children in State X ages 12-17 considered by others to have a disability?
a. What is the expected number of children in State X ages 0-17 considered by others to have fair to poor health?

Exercise 5
Estimating various disability measures controlling
for one other factor (poverty status)

Table 6 provides a sample of measures from previous tables controlling for poverty. Table 2 contains summary population data for State X.

Use information from Table 2 and Table 6 to answer the following questions:

a. What is the expected number of children in State X ages 0-17, adjusting for poverty status, with an activity limitation?
b. What is the expected number of children in State X ages 0-17, adjusting for poverty status, considered by others to have fair or poor health?

Exercise 6
Developing a combined estimate for disability

Table 7 provides two tables generated directly from the *SETS* program of two mutually exclusive estimates of disability.

Table 8 provides a combined estimate using data from Table 7.

Table 2 contains summary population data for State X

Use information from Table 2 and Table 8 to answer the following questions:

a. What is the expected number of children in State X ages 0-17 with activity limitation or fair or poor health?

Code book names used by NCHS for measures used in this module
(1994 National Health Interview Survey on Disability, Phase 1)

Measure	Variable name
Learning disability	LEARNR
Mental retardation	RETARDR
Cerebral palsy	CERPALSR
Muscular dystrophy	MUSCDYSR
Spina bifida	SPNBIFR
Cystic Fibrosis	CYSFIBR
Activity limitation	LATOTAL
Difficulty with strenuous activity	DIFSTACT
Goes to the doctor or specialist regularly	REGDR
Receives therapy in or out of the home	TXHOME12=yes or TXSCHOOL=yes
Respondent considers person to have a disability	RPPERDIS
Respondent considers this person to have fair or poor health	HEALTH = fair or poor

Table 1
Summary data describing the prevalence of specific conditions amongst children under age 18

(1994 National Health Interview Survey on Disability, Phase 1)

Characteristic	All ages 17 years and under	0-5 years	6-11 years	12-17 years
All Children	70,023,660	24,507,881	23,196,284	22,319,495
Learning Disability	2,284,385 (3.3%)	148,401 (0.6%)	1,014,431 (4.4%)	1,121,553 (5%)
Mental Retardation	242,877 (0.3%)	44,356 (0.2%)	92,917 (0.4%)	105,604 (0.5%)
Cerebral Palsy	136,913 (0.2%)	42,972 (0.2%)	61,281 (0.3%)	32,660 (0.1%)
Muscular Dystrophy	21,518 (0.03%)	----	12,768 (0.06%)	8,750 (0.04%)
Spina Bifida	19,783 (0.03%)	----	13,140 (0.06%)	6,643 (0.03%)
Cystic Fibrosis	10,955 (0.02%)	4,950 (0.02%)	6,005 (0.03%)	---

-- no one identified in the group

Note: for conditions only the Yes and No responses applied to percents; "not ascertained or refused" were not included

Table 2
Census Data for State X on Selected Demographic Characteristics

(1994 Census, Summary Tape File 3A.)

Characteristic	Number	Percent
Total Population		
Ages 0-17	2,946,365	----
Ages 0-5	1,018,444	34.6%
Ages 6-11	1,211,253	41.1%
Ages 12-17	716,668	24.3%
Poverty Status		
Ages 0-17 at or above poverty	2,450,860	83.2%
Ages 0-17 below poverty	495,505	16.8%
Ages 0-5 at or above poverty	254,785	25.0%

Table 3
Summary data describing functional limitations amongst children under age 18

(1994 National Health Interview Survey on Disability, Phase 1.)

Characteristic	All ages 17 ages and un-der	0-5 years	6-11 years	12-17 years
All Children	70,023,660	24,507,881	23,196,284	22,319,495
Activity Status				
Not Limited	65,279,818 (93.2%)	23,676,885 (96.6%)	21,262,861 (91.7%)	20,340,072 (91.1%)
Limited	4,743,842 (6.7%)	830,996 (3.4%)	1,933,423 (8.3%)	1,979,423 (8.9%)
Difficulty with Strenuous Activity	1,756,150 (2.5%)	272,141 (1.1%)	638,148 (2.8%)	845,861 (3.8%)

Table 4
Summary data describing health service utilization
amongst children under age 18

(1994 National Health Interview Survey on Disability, Phase 1)

Characteristics	All ages 17 years and under	0-5 years	6-11 years	12-17 years
All Children	70,023,660	24,507,881	23,196,284	22,319,495
Goes to the doctor or specialist on a regular basis	44,018,816 (5.7%)	858,353 (4.2%)	1,459,995(6.3%)	1,524,401 (6.8%)
Receives therapy in or out of the home	475,129 (0.7%)	198,195 (0.8%)	179,680 (0.8%)	48,776 (0.3%)

Table 5
Summary data describing perception of disability
amongst children under age 18

(1994 National Health Interview Survey on Disability, Phase 1)

Characteristics	All ages 17 years and under	0-5 years	6-11 years	12-17 years
All Children	70,023,660	24,507,881	23,196,284	22,319,495
Respondent considers this person to have a disability	1,724,343 (2.5%)	236,801 (1.2%)	705,498 (3%)	708,573 (3.2%)
Respondent considers this person to have fair or poor health	2,013,723 (2.9%)	564,386 (2.8%)	682,617 (2.9%)	663,207 (3.0%)

Table 6
Summary data describing various measures for children under age 18

(1994 National Health Interview Survey on Disability, Phase 1)

Characteris-tics	All ages 17 years and under	At or above poverty	Below poverty
All Children	70,023,660	52, 304,455 (74.7%)	13,062,688 (18.7%)
Learning Disability	2,284,385 (3.3%)	1,576,074 (3%)	545,828 (4.2%)
Has an activity limitation	4,743,842 (6.7%)	3,085,866 (5.8%)	1,284,540 (9.9%)
Goes to the doctor or specialist on a regular basis	44,018,816 (5.7%)	3,165,330 (6.1%)	636,664 (4.9%)
Respondent considers this person to have fair or poor health	2,013,723 (2.9%)	1,035,694 (2%)	750,174 (5.7%)

* The poverty category 'unknown' is not shown in table, therefore the numbers in the last two columns do not total to the figures in column "All ages 17 years and under."

Table 7
Tables from the NHIS on Disability, Phase 1, Using *SETS*

LATOTAL/LABELS	
File: PERSON.DAT	
Records: Age<18	
Weight: WTFA	
LATOTAL	70023660.00
Unable to perform major activity	505274.00
Limited in kind/amount major activity	2975491.00
Limited in other activities	1263077.00
Not limited (includes unknowns)	65279818.00

HEALTH/LABELS	
File: PERSON.DAT	
Records: Age<18 AND LATOTAL=4 (or not limited)	
Weight: WTFA	
HEALTH	65279818.00
Excellent	34724617.00
Very Good	17909337.00
Good	10672016.00
Fair	1044213.00
Poor	89065.00
Unknown	840570.00

Table 8
Estimates of children with activity limitations and fair or poor health combined

Children with activity limitations:
= All children - not limited
= 70,023,660 - 65,279,818 = 4,743,842 (6.8%)

Children with fair or poor health:
= fair health + poor health
= 1,044,213 + 89,065 = 1,133,278

Children who are activity limited OR have fair or poor health:
= children activity limited + other children in fair or poor health
= 4,743,842 + 1,133,278 = 5,877,120 (8.4%)

Solutions

Exercise 1a

$0.006 \times 1{,}018{,}444$
$=6{,}110$

Exercise 1b

$0.002 \times 2{,}946{,}365$
$=5{,}893$

Exercise 2a

$0.038 \times 716{,}668$
$=27{,}233$

Exercise 2b

$0.067 \times 2{,}946{,}365$
$=197{,}406$

Exercise 3a

$0.068 \times 716{,}668$
$=48{,}733$

Exercise 3b

$0.007 \times 2{,}946{,}365$
$=20{,}624$

Exercise 4a

$0.032 \times 716{,}668$
$=22{,}933$

Exercise 4b

$0.029 \times 2{,}946{,}365$
$=85{,}445$

Exercise 5a

At or above poverty $=142{,}150$
Below poverty $=49{,}055$
Adjusted total $=191{,}205$
{Crude total $=197{,}406$}

Exercise 5b

At or above poverty $=49{,}017$
Below poverty $=28{,}244$
Adjusted total $=77{,}262$
{Crude total $=85{,}445$}

Exercise 6

$0.084 \times 2{,}946{,}365$
$=247{,}495$

References

Eyman, R.K., H.J. Grossman, R.H. Chaney, and T.L. Call. 1990. "The Life Expectancy of Profoundly Handicapped People with Mental Retardation." *The New England Journal of Medicine* 323(9): 584-589.

Hogan, D.P., M.E. Msall, M.L. Rogers, and R. Avery. 1997. "Improved population estimates of functional limitation among American children age 5-17". Presentation at NCHS.

McManus, M. 1997. "Defining and identifying children with special health care needs." Presented at the Children with Special Health Care Needs Institute (October 29, 1997), Columbus, Ohio.

Muldoon, J.H., J.M. Neff, J.C. Gay. 1997. "Profiling the health service needs of populations using diagnosis-based classification systems." *The Journal of Ambulatory Care Management* 20(3).

National Institute of Health/NICHD. 1993. Research Plan for the National Center on Medical Rehabilitation Research. NIH Publication No. 93-3509.

Newacheck, P. and W. Taylor. 1992. "Childhood Chronic Illness: Prevalence, Severity, and Impact." *American Journal of Public Health* 82(3): 364-71.

Stein, R.E.K., L.J. Bauman, L.E. Westbrook, S.M. Coupey, and H.T. Ireys. 1993. "Framework for identifying children who have chronic conditions: The case for a new definition." *The Journal of Pediatrics* 122: 42-347.

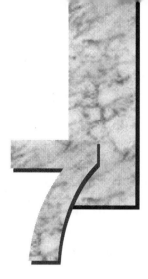

Using Census Data in MCH

by Colleen Monahan, DC, MPH

Public health policy decisions and needs assessments are predicated on interpretations and conclusions drawn from combining the results from many individuals or a population. The use of current estimates of population characteristics is necessary to make estimates of disease, injury, disability, behaviors of interest to public health, and their distributions. Often, these estimates require population denominators from the census.

This module outlines the history of the census in the United States and its use as a source of data for MCH planning or analysis. Much analysis and reporting of public health data relies on knowledge of the use of census data. This module provides background information required to use census data.

This module will address:

- Description of the census
- History of the census
- Evolution of the U.S. census
- Census in the Year 2000
- The modern census
- Census content and sample design
- Problems and limitations of census estimates
- Census geography
- Dissemination of census products
- Uses of census data for demographic and socioeconomic analysis
- Summary of technical issues for calculating totals and percents using census data

DESCRIPTION OF THE CENSUS

The decennial census provides us basic information on the number of persons and their demographic, socioeconomic, and household characteristics. Since our activities in public health must be predicated on a count of the population to be served, this census data supplies us with the denominators for our morbidity and mortality rates. It also provides us with count data that we may use when applying rates and proportions obtained on various issues from national or state surveys. For example, the state Behavioral Risk Factor Survey identified that 20% of households with children had an adult who smoked cigarettes. If a local community wanted to target households with children as their first cut in an anti-smoking program, they would use census data to obtain the total number of households with children and calculate 20% of them to be the number they would target for the program.

Census data can be used to support MCH planning by:

- identifying estimates for the total number of persons eligible for a particular program (target population) and the subsequent calculation of program coverage (number served divided by the target population estimate);
- identifying risk markers for adverse behaviors or health outcomes, e.g., poverty status, occupation, and so forth;
- developing indices by combining risk factors (e.g., the rate of single-parent households living in poverty combined with the proportion of families living in poverty); and,
- comparing the characteristics of a community to the state or to other communities.

HISTORY OF THE CENSUS

MCH data analysis for planning and programming rely upon knowledge of the size and composition of a population and the census provides us with a valuable source of population-based data. The census provides data on the population, socioeconomic, and housing characteristics of the entire country and affects our lives in three major areas: political power, federal and state program funding distribution, and planning activities.

In the United States, the census of population has been conducted every ten years, beginning in 1790. Originally, this enumeration was the result of a political compromise arising from the conflict between sparsely populated states and heavily populated states. The former wanted equal representation in the national legislature, while the latter believed that their larger populations justified greater power. The compromise was the establishment of our bicameral legislature in which the states are equally represented in the Senate and are represented according to population size in the House of Representatives. Since the House seats are apportioned according to the size of the population, it is necessary for a periodic inventory of the population. This periodic inventory required by the United States Constitution. Article I, Section 2, Paragraph 3 (Modified by the Fourteenth Amendment) calls for the enumeration of the country's population every ten years. The results of this constitutionally required enumeration determine not only the apportionment of House seats, but influence how the boundaries for congressional and state legislative districts are drawn. Additionally, at the county and municipal levels, election districts must be drawn using census statistics to ensure equal representation.

Census data are used by the Federal and state governments to allocate billions of dollars every year to the local governments for a wide variety of public purposes, including the allocation of State MCH Block Grant funds. Since public health initiatives are greatly affected by Federal and state funding, an understanding of how census data are collected, as well as the uses and limitations of the data, is important.

The Evolution of the U.S. Census

While the original census included only three questions: color, free or slave status and the sex of free white persons, the United States census (http://www.census.gov/) has evolved to encompass data on other characteristics about the population as well as housing. Census surveys have also been developed to monitor economic activities. There are census surveys of agriculture, wholesale and retail trade, services industries, construction industries, manufacturers, mineral industries, and transportation. Public and private agencies and corporations use census data for such diverse purposes as marketing, analysis of social and economic trends and estimating the magnitude of the target population size for program planning.

The Census Bureau was established in 1902 to oversee the census. Bureau staff generate questions that are reviewed by the Bureau Director and the Office of Management and Budget (OMB). The Congress must be advised of proposed topics to the Census three years prior to the actual enumeration. Two years prior to the enumeration Congress must be provided with the wording of the proposed questions. The Bureau solicits input for questions by conducting local public meetings throughout the United States. Diverse ethnic groups and minority populations are consulted about question content and wording. The Bureau also solicits information on the level of aggregation of various data that should be made available. In addition to defining what information is to be collected, the Bureau also defines what information may not be collected on the country's population. Religious affiliation and Social Security Numbers are two examples of such taboo variables. Though standards exist to maintain the privacy of those being enumerated, data from the census can be and has been misused. Most notably, census data were used during the Civil War to identify the number of free and slave African-Americans prior to General Sherman's March to the Sea campaign and during World War II to identify the location of Japanese-Americans in the United States.

The 1990 Census

Revisions to the 1990 Census of Population and Housing reflect the larger changes in American society. For example, evolving family structure brought many changes to the census description of the relationship of children to adults in the surveyed household. Terms such as stepson, stepdaughter, grandchild, foster child, and unmarried partner were included for the first time in the 1990 Census. While the race category still includes "Black or Negro" and Spanish/Hispanic," "Other" could be written-in in the 1990 Census. American Indian tribes and Pacific Islander groups were delineated for the first time, resulting in a large increase in the percentage of American Indians reported in the 1990 Census. Unlike the 1980 Census, in 1990 the question regarding educational attainment was included on the long form questionnaire (received by 1 of 6 households), rather than on the short form (received by 100 percent of households.) (The distinctions between the two versions of the forms will be described later in the module). The disability status of adult persons in the household was also included for the first time in the 1990 Census.

The census with which most of us are familiar and to which we have referred to directly above, is known as the Decennial Census of Population and Housing. This census includes several data items or variables that are of particular interest and use in a public health setting. These variables include total persons, households, families, age, race, and ethnicity, poverty (as defined as the minimum level of acceptable subsistence income of a family or household), and income to poverty ratio.

Population and housing data are also tracked with surveys between the Decennial Census. The *Current Population Survey* (CPS) (http://www.bls.census.gov/cps/cpsmain.htm) helps identify intercensal year growth and migration of populations as well as monitor socioeconomic trends. Estimates obtained from the CPS include employment, unemployment, earnings, hours of work, and other indicators. They are available by a variety of demographic characteristics including age, sex, race, marital status, and educational attainment. They are also available by occupation, industry, and class of worker. Supplemental questions to produce estimates on a variety of topics including school enrollment, income, previous work experience, health, employee benefits, and work schedules are also often added to the regular CPS questionnaire.

The *Survey on Income and Program Participation* (SIPP) (http://www.census.gov/hhes/sippdesc.html) tracks information on persons participating in federal financial entitlement programs, such as Supplemental Social Security (SSI), Medicare, and Medicaid. The sample design for the first SIPP panel in 1984 consisted of about 20,000 households selected to represent the noninstitutional population of the United States. The most recent 1993 panel has a sample size of approximately 20,000 households. Households in this SIPP panel are scheduled to be interviewed at four-month intervals over a period of 3 years.

Census in the Year 2000

The Year 2000 census will be changing. The Census 2000 operational plan redesigns the census process in bold and fundamental ways. Go to the Internet census site to keep abreast of all these changes at the following address: http://www.census.gov/dmd/www/plan2.html or review the plan that the Census Bureau disseminated at the time this document was written.

The Modern Census

A modern census has four key elements. It should be:

1. Universal
2. Simultaneous
3. Periodic
4. Individual

For a census to be *universal*, it must include everyone in the population being enumerated. Problems arise when attempting to count the homeless, minority males in poverty, and Native Americans, since these groups may not be living in conventional settings that are more easily enumerated.

There are two methods for enumerating a population: *de facto,* which allocates persons according to their location at the time of enumeration; and *de jure*, which assigns persons according to their usual place of residence. The United States uses a de jure enumeration because it provides a better indication of the permanent population and household composition of an area. For example, a professor who lives in Kenosha, Wisconsin may actually teach at a university in Chicago. On the day of a de facto census, she would be assigned to Chicago. If a de jure census were used, she would be assigned to Kenosha. Census forms should be mailed *simultaneously* to people at their usual place of residence. The return date for the forms should be the same for everyone; however, some forms are returned late and individuals are sometimes interviewed after the official due date.

A census should be *periodic*. Counts should be made at regular intervals. As discussed earlier, the United States Constitution sets the frequency of our census at every ten years. The Census is now conducted as of April 30 of every Decennial census year.

Finally, in a modern census, the individual is counted and described. In the past, women and slaves, for example, were not enumerated as individuals, but as belonging to the white, male head of the household.

CENSUS CONTENT AND SAMPLE DESIGN

When preparing for the Decennial Census of Population and Housing, the Census Bureau compiles and checks an address list of approximately 106 million housing units and approximately 250 million people across the United States. The Census Bureau is also responsible for enumerating people and housing units in Puerto Rico, the Virgin Islands of the United States, Guam, the Commonwealth of the Northern Mariana Islands, American Samoa, and Palau. This entire population receives a short form, while one of every six households also receives a long form. In both cases, one individual in each household completes the information for the entire household. These two forms are described below.

Short Form

The short form is intended for surveying 100% of the population, an estimated 106 million households. This form, completed by all households, includes:

- seven population questions applicable to every individual in the household; and
- seven questions concerning the household's housing conditions.

Data are available on Summary Tape File 1 for all the short form responses at every geographic level known to the census. You may view the tables available or locate tables by subject.

Data collected from this form are contained in Summary Tape File 1 (STF1) and Summary Tape File 2 (STF2). The Summary Tape Files will be discussed in detail later in this module.

Long Form

Completed by approximately 17.7 million households, the long form includes information about place of birth, participation in the labor force, and family income. The long form survey is conducted on a sample of the U.S. population. The sampling rates vary, depending on geographic locations and population size. The purpose of using variable sampling rates is to provide relatively more reliable estimates for small areas and decrease respondent burden in more densely populated areas while maintaining data reliability. Higher proportions of less populous areas receive the long form. For example, locations with less than 2,500 persons sample one in two households, while locations with more than 2,500 persons sample one in six households. Some densely populated areas sample one in eight.

Summary Tape File 3 (STF 3) and Summary Tape File 4 (STF4) contain the data collected from these long forms. You may view the tables available or locate tables by subject.

When working with census data, it is important to remember the distinctions between the short and the long forms. Variations between the two formats include the:

- geographic area summarized;
- topics covered; and
- media format in which the data can be accessed.

When designing the census questionnaire, the Bureau tries to include questions that allow for comparison with previous census data, questions of current interest to lawmakers as well as special interest groups, and questions that people will willingly answer, i.e., questions that do not make people feel their privacy is being invaded. The tables below list the data items that were collected in the 1990 Census.

100-Percent Component (Short Form)

POPULATION	HOUSING
Household relationship Sex Race Age Marital status Hispanic origin	Number of units in structure Number of rooms in units Tenure-owned or rented Value of home or monthly rent Congregate housing (meals included in rent) Vacancy characteristics

Sample Component (Long Form)

POPULATION	HOUSING
Social Characteristics	
Education-enrollment and attainment Place of birth, citizenship, and year of entry into U.S. Ancestry Language spoken at home Migration (residence in 1985) Disability Fertility Veteran status	Year moved into residence Number of bedrooms Plumbing and kitchen facilities Telephone in unit Vehicles available Heating fuel Source of water and method of sewage disposal Year structure built Condominium status Farm residence Shelter costs, including utilities
Economic Characteristics	
Labor force participation Occupation, industry, and class of worker Work experience in 1989 Income in 1989 Year last worked	

CENSUS GEOGRAPHY

Understanding the geographic components of the census is crucial when we are using census data. Since many of our planning and programming decisions are based on political or legal definitions of a region or area, we need to be aware of the geography by which census data are reported. For example, one can estimate population denominators for city-based data (a political area) using the census but in order to examine the city by smaller geographic areas statistical area data must be examined (e.g., block, census tracts, etc.). Political and statistical areas are not subsets of each other. Although a large city may be composed of multiple census tracts, tracts near the city borders would overlap those borders. Special algorithms must be developed when attempting to combine data from political and statistical areas. One area of geography not considered in census geography are postal codes or zip codes. The Census Bureau does report data in STF3 by zip code but does not collect data by this geographic level. In addition, zip code level data are reported at least a couple of years post release of other census data.

Following is a description of the political and the statistical areas as defined by the Census Bureau.

Political areas include:

- The United States
- Individual states, the District of Columbia, Puerto Rico, the Virgin Islands of the United States, Guam, the Commonwealth of the Northern Mariana Islands, American Samoa, and Palau
- Congressional districts
- Counties
- Minor civil divisions (MCDs) i.e., legal subdivisions of counties, called townships in many states
- Incorporated places, e.g., cities, villages, and so forth
- American Indian reservations and associated trust lands
- Alaska Native Regional Corporations (ANRCs)

Statistical areas include:

- *Census regions and divisions*: the 50 states and the District of Columbia have been grouped into four regions: Northeast, North Central, South, and West, each containing two or three divisions, e.g., New England, Middle Atlantic. There are a total of nine divisions.

- *Metropolitan Statistical Areas (MSAs),* formerly known as Standard Metropolitan Statistical Areas (SMSAs): Areas consisting of one or more counties, including a large population nucleus and nearby communities that have a high degree of interaction. *Primary metropolitan statistical areas (PMSAs) are MSAs that make up consolidated metropolitan statistical areas (CMSAs).*

- *Urbanized Areas (UAs):* Defined by population density, each includes a central city and the surrounding closely settled urban fringe (suburbs) that together have a population of 50,000 or more with a population density generally exceeding 1,000 per square mile.

- *Urban/Rural:* All persons living in urbanized area and in places of 2,500 or more population outside of UAs constitute the "urban" population; all others constitute the rural population.

- *Census County Divisions:* Statistical subdivisions of a county defined by the Census Bureau in cooperation with state officials in 21 states where minor civil divisions do not exist or are not adequate for producing subcounty statistics.

- *Census Designated Places (CDPs):* Densely settled population centers without legally defined corporate limits or corporate powers.

- *Census Tracts:* Small, locally defined statistical areas in metropolitan areas and some other counties. They generally have stable boundaries and an average population of 4,000.

- *Block Numbering Areas (BNAs):* Areas defined, with state assistance, for grouping and numbering blocks and reporting statistics in counties without census tracts.

- *Block Groups:* Groupings of census blocks within census tracts and BNAs. These replace the enumeration districts or EDs for which the Census Bureau provided data for many areas of the country in the 1980 census.

- *Blocks:* The smallest census geographic areas, normally bounded by streets and other prominent physical features. County, MCD, and place limits also serve as block boundaries. Blocks may be as small as a typical city block bounded by four streets or as large as several square miles in rural areas. The 1990 census was the first census in which data were available by block for the entire country.

- *Alaska Native Village Statistical Areas (ANVSAs):* A 1990 census statistical area that delineates the settled area of each Alaska Native village (ANV). Officials of the Alaska Native Regional Corporations (business and nonprofit corporate entities) outlined the ANVSAs for the Census Bureau for the sole purpose of presenting 1990 census data.

- *Tribal Designated Statistical Areas (TDSAs):* Geographic areas outlined for 1990 census tabulations purposes by American Indian tribal officials of recognized tribes that do not have a recognized land area.

- *Tribal Jurisdiction Statistical Areas (TJSAs):* Geographic areas delineated by tribal officials in Oklahoma for the 1990 census tabulation purposes.

DISSEMINATION OF CENSUS PRODUCTS

The Census Bureau disseminates their products (http://www.census.gov/mp/www/censtore.html) in a variety of formats, including non-print formats. Traditional formats include printed reports and maps, as well as computer tape. The Bureau also releases a number of products on microfiche and CD-ROM laser disks, as well as through its online service, CENDATA™. Information is also disseminated through Topographically Integrated Geographic Encoding and Referencing (TIGER).

Printed Reports

Census data contained in the printed reports are arranged in tables; population and housing characteristics are presented for specified geographic areas. The 1990 Census printed report series presented data at the small-area level, such as census tracts; only limited subject-matter detail is included. For example, counts of individuals were reported by age groups, less than 5 years, 5 to 9 years, and so forth, rather than by single years.

Computer Tapes

Decennial Census data have been available on computer tapes since the 1960 Census. The Census Bureau provides much more data on computer tape than in its printed reports. For example, all of the tabulated figures appear on the computer tapes. This is not true of the printed reports. Computer tapes provide census statistics in more detail than is available in the printed reports. These tapes are particularly useful if we need to manipulate, aggregate, or plan any extensive processing of the data.

Summary Tape Files (STFs)

Mentioned briefly in our discussion of the long and the short forms, summary tape files are designed to provide statistics with greater subject detail for geographic areas than is feasible in printed reports. The STFs contain the same types of information available in the reports, but there is more information available. There were four STFs produced for the 1990 Census. Each of these four summary tape files contains specific types of data. The figure below highlights the important features of each STF:

Main Features of Summary Tape Files

	STF1	STF2	STF3	STF4
100-Percent Data	X	X		
Sample Data		X	X	
Presents a particular set of data tables for specific types of geographic areas	X	X	X	X
Contains 3 or more file types that differ in the types of geographic detail reported, but contain the same detail.	X	X	X	X
1990 STF comparable to 1980 STFs	X	X	X	X

STFs 1 and 3 will have more geograhic levels detailed, but less data detail than STFs 2 and 4.

STF 5, released in 1980 for the United States, each state, and the District of Columbia, was not issued in 1990. Comparable data provided through the 1990 subject reports and related STFs is discussed below.

Technical documentation guides contain an abstract describing the type of file, the subject matter, and the geographic coverage of the data contained on each STF. The guides also provide valuable information on how to use the files, how information is segmented and coded, as well as numerous appendices containing information such as code lists, facsimiles of respondent instructions and questionnaire pages, collections and processing procedures, and a description of the accuracy of the data.

Public Use Microdata Samples (PUMs)

Public Use Microdata Sample Files (PUMs) (http://www.census.gov/ftp/pub/mp/www/rom/msrom6h.html) are microdata files on computer tape that present a sample of unidentified long-form housing-unit records for large geographic areas. Each housing-unit sample record presents essentially all the census data collected about each person in a sample household, plus the housing unit's characteristics. This is the only method available for tabulating information on all members within a household. The other census files have information on individuals or households, but there is no way to make informational links between household members.

There are two sets of public use microdata files (PUMs): a five- percent sample and a one- percent sample. The five- percent sample is grouped by counties or county groups that do not cross state boundaries and includes at least 100,000 persons. Codes are included that indicate to the user in what group of counties or area the household is located.

The one percent sample also includes at least 100,000 persons, but is organized by metropolitan area and may cross states boundaries.

The PUMs allows users with special needs to prepare customized tabulations and cross-tabulations of virtually any item on the census questionnaire.

Other Special Computer Tape Files

Other computer tape files include the *Public Law (PL) 94-171 Counts File*. The Public Law Counts File is released before the regular Census files to allow political boundaries to be drawn in each state. This file contains statistics on total population, age, race, Hispanic origin, while the EEO File contains sample tabulations showing detailed occupations and educational attainment by age. This file is cross-tabulated by sex, Hispanic origin, and race. The Migration File contains summary statistics for all intra-state county-to-county migration streams and significant inter-state county-to-county migration streams.

Microfiche

In the 1990 Census, block statistics were available on microfiche. The microfiche presented a subset of the tabulations for blocks found on STF1B. As mentioned previously, 1990 was the first time the entire country was blocked. This served to increase the number of blocks for which the Census Bureau provided data from 2.5 million in 1980 to approximately 7 million in 1990. The microfiche format allows for the storage of the vast quantities of data. The cost and storage of this block data would be prohibitive in a printed report format. STFs 1A and 3A are available on microfiche.

CD-ROM

The CD-ROM format is another technology that allows for the cost- and space-efficient storage of large amounts of data. The 1990 Census data available on CD-ROM included the *Public Law (PL) 94-171* tape file and STFs 1-3. We can expect to see an increasing number of data files to be made available on CD-ROM for the year 2000 Census.

Special Tabulations

The Census Bureau, for a fee, will prepare special tabulations for any specific geographic or subject matter area. Standard reports, tapes, and microfiche should be used whenever possible, since special tabulations are expensive and are only done when the Bureau staff has completed their regular work.

Online Services

The Census Bureau (http://www.census.gov) maintains a comprehensive web site where links exist to the following data sites:

CenStats and CenStore are located at: http://www.census.gov/mp/www/index2.html
Tiger file mapping service can be found at: http://tiger.census.gov/
1990 census data lookup can be accessed: http://venus.census.gov/cdrom/lookup

Maps and Geographic Files

Census maps are vital for all users of small-area census data. Additionally, census maps are needed to locate specific geographic areas and show the spatial relationship of the data. Among the maps available for the 1990 Census were:

County Block Maps: details the census blocks and their numbers, other boundaries, and physical features.

County Subdivisions Maps: presents the boundaries of the counties, county subdivisions (MCDs or CCDs), places, American Indian reservations, including off-reservation trust lands, and the Alaska Native areas.

Census Tract/BNA Outline Maps: depicts the census tract/block numbering area (BNA) boundaries and features underlying the boundaries.

Machine-Readable Geographic Files

The Census Bureau developed an automated geographic database, known as TIGER or Topologically Integrated Geographic and Encoding and Referencing. This system allows for the production of various geographic products that support the census data. It also provides coordinate-based digital map information for the entire United States, the Virgin Islands of the United States, and the Pacific territories. The TIGER System allows us to create computer-generated maps at different scales for any geographic are of the country. TIGER System extracts are available in several formats, including TIGER/Line files. TIGER/Line Files is a file with selected geographic and cartographic information containing basic data for the segments of each boundary or feature; including:

- adjacent census geographic area codes;
- latitude and longitude coordinates of segment end points;
- the name and type of feature; the relevant census feature class code identifying the feature segment by category; and,
- address ranges and associated zip codes for both sides of the street segments for areas approximating the urbanized areas.

TIGER/Line files are organized by county and are available on computer tape and CD-ROM.

USES OF CENSUS DATA FOR DEMOGRAPHIC AND SOCIOECOMONIC ANALYSIS

Demographics

Demographic data from the census can be used to describe the racial and ethnic characteristics of an area. Racial and ethnic data are given for the total population, and then for the population by age categories zero through seventeen. Racial categories are white, black, American Indian, Eskimo, or Aleutian or Pacific Islander, and other races. Remember that racial categories do *not* include Hispanic, since

Hispanics include black, white, and other races. Hispanics are identified as an ethnic group by the U.S. census, and are subdivided into Mexican, Puerto Rican, Cuban, and other Hispanic. Ethnic origin refers to Hispanic origin only, and does not include people of other European, Asian, or African ethnicities, e.g. Irish, Japanese, or Kenyan.

The numbers and percents for the racial categories for any group given in the demographics section (i.e., total population, population ages zero through two, population ages three through five, etc.) should add up to 100 percent. The ethnic or Hispanic origin numbers and percents are *not* related to the racial numbers and percents. Do not add Hispanic numbers or percents to racial numbers or percents.

Census data tells us that the population of minority groups in the United States has been growing over the past decades, especially in the last ten years, due in part to immigration and a higher fertility rates among these groups. Demographers indicate that minority populations will continue to grow over the next two decades. Minority populations are disproportionately disadvantaged in terms of family income, access to health care, access to high-quality education, and employment opportunities. We can use demographic numbers from the census as denominators when calculating percents of people served by particular programs as a percent of total number of people in a certain age or racial group.

The measurement of race is being changed through the Office of Management and Budget (OMB) which released new guidelines to OMB Directive 15 in July 1997. Developed in 1977, the original Directive 15 describes four races (Native American or Alaskan Native; Asian or Pacific Islander; Black; and White) and two ethnic categories (of Hispanic origin and not of Hispanic origin). Although the Directive notes the absence of scientific or anthropological foundations in its formulation, race and ethnic categories are used in federal scientific research and, as such, serve as a basis for interpreting research findings, ranging from biomedical to economic research. However, race and ethnicity categories used by the census have changed over time and rely upon an inconsistent mixture of principles and criteria, including national origin, language, minority status and physical characteristics. Since 1900, 26 different racial terms have been used to identify populations on the US Census.

The concept of race is a social and cultural construction, with no basis in human biology. Race can simply not be tested or proven scientifically, according to the American Anthropological Association (AAA). In addition, many Americans do not understand differences between race, ethnicity and ancestry categories in surveys, and fail to distinguish between them. The new OMB Directive will change the way the Year 2000 census defines race and present new challenges for analysis and trending of data.

Socioeconomic Data

Socioeconomic data available from the census include children living in poverty by age groups, single-householder families living in poverty, children living in households with unemployed parents, number of adults with a high school education, unemployment figures for an area, and the primary language spoken in the home.

Socioeconomic data are important to public health analysis because certain socioeconomic data are strong risk markers, or indicators, for unfavorable health outcomes such as low birth weight, child neglect and abuse, and teenage pregnancy.

To understand the socioeconomic data from the U.S. census, we need to understand how the census defines several key terms-household, householder, family, and related child.

Household—all the persons who occupy a housing unit.

Householder—In most cases, a householder is the person, or one of the persons, in whose name the home is owned, being bought, or rented, or any adult household member fifteen years old or over designated as the householder for purposes of the census.

Family—-a householder and one or more other persons living in the same household who are related to the householder by birth, marriage, or adoption. All persons in a household who are related to the householder are regarded as members of his or her family. A household can contain only one family for purposes of the census.

Related child—a son or daughter by birth, a stepchild, or an adopted child. The term does not include foster children.

Socioeconomic Indicators

Examples of socioeconomic risk markers or indicators of unfavorable health outcomes for children, and why they are important to consider in a public health analysis are described below.

Poverty
Although the mean income of families with children has risen over the last thirty years—due to an increase in family income and a decrease in the average number of children per family, more families with children than ever before are economically insecure. Today, one in five children in the United States lives in a family below the federal poverty level. Nationwide, almost 13 million children live in poverty, more than 2 million more than ten years ago. Of these children, almost 5 million live in families with incomes less than half the federal poverty level. Minority children are much more likely to live in a poor family. Children living in a single-parent family, especially if that parent is a mother, are likely to be poor.

Children in poor families in economically disadvantaged neighborhoods have the most health and behavioral problems. These children have lower literacy levels and higher rates of dropping out of high school. They have a greater exposure to violence. Poverty affects access to health care and availability of services and has been linked with higher levels of child neglect and abuse.

Single-householder families
Children growing up in families with one parent are more likely to be poor than children in families with two parents. When the single parent is a mother, the risk factor for poverty increases. Nationwide, about 43 percent of single-mother families live below poverty, compared to only about 7 percent of two-parent families. If the mothers are not working, these children are very likely to be poor. While poverty among two-parent families usually fluctuates with the economy, poverty among single-mother families remains constant; among these families, sustained poverty for seven or more years is common, whereas this is rare for two-parent families. The average income of single-mother families is only about 40 percent of the average income of two-parent families at the same age. The economic status of single-mother families is often exacerbated by the failure of absent fathers to pay child support.

Single-householder families living below poverty with children under age five
This is a combination of two major socioeconomic risk factors.

Children living with one or two parents and all parents are unemployed
When no parents are unemployed in a family with children, the children are at even more risk for the unfavorable outcomes associated with poverty, listed above.

SUMMARY OF TECHNICAL ISSUES FOR CALCULATING TOTALS AND PERCENTS USING CENSUS DATA

To make use of census data, an understanding of file organization is important. This discussion will be limited to the data found on the CR-ROM version of the STFs, discussed earlier in this module. The CD-ROM is packaged with browsing software called "GO" that was developed by the Census Bureau to simplify retrieval of summary tables. Once the CD is in the drive, all the user has to do to start the program is type: GO. You may then select the geographic area of interest and then the data item of interest. The data are stored in the CD-ROM in a database format. When copying the data for use elsewhere, the user is given the options of database field (*.dbf) and ASCII (delimited or fixed). It is important to note that a single data item selected (such as poverty by age) is stored as a separate database table and each group you see displayed is a separate variable in the data table. Therefore, in the case of poverty by age, if you want to create a variable for number and percent of persons under age 18 under poverty you would need to sum each age variable (0-4, 5, 6-13, and so forth) that makes up the total number of persons under 18 years.

Careful attention must be paid to calculating the denominator you will use to obtain your percent variable. Each database table has a universe of values, e.g., persons on whom the data were obtained, households, families, and so forth. For example, if a table describes the universe as being "persons greater than or equal to age 25" then the denominator used for any variable within the table must be the total number of persons greater than or equal to age 25. This variable may be obtained by creating a total for all categories in the table or through totaling the number of persons in the age group using the table for age. The totals between the tables may or may not match. This may be due to suppression or other reasons unknown to this author. In either case, the safest method is to use the total for the table that was the source of the numerator.

Exercises: Using Census Data in MCH

Refer to the electronic version of this workbook for exercises in *Using Census Data in MCH*.

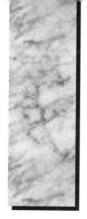

SUMMARY OF
COMMONLY USED FORMULAE

1. Prevalence and Incidence

Prevalence Rate

$$= \frac{\text{\# of individuals with a health condition}}{\text{\# individuals in the relevant population}} \text{ at a given point in time}$$

Cumulative Incidence Rate

$$= \frac{\text{\# of new cases of a health outcome during a given period of time}}{\text{\# at risk of developing the outcome at the start of the period}}$$

Incidence Density

$$= \frac{\text{\# new cases of a health outcome}}{\text{Total person time of observation}} \text{ during a given period of time}$$

2. Statistical Estimation

$$\text{Accuracy} = \text{Bias} + \text{Reliability}$$

Means, proportions, and rates are all averages:

$$E(\overline{X}) = \mu \quad \text{and} \quad \overline{X} = \frac{\sum_{i=1}^{n} X_i}{n}, \quad E(p) = \pi \quad \text{and} \quad p = \frac{\sum_{i=1}^{n} X_i}{n}, \quad E(r) = \lambda \quad \text{and} \quad r = \frac{\sum_{i=1}^{n} X_i}{n}$$

The standard deviation is a measure of the average deviation of *individual observations* around their mean:

$$\text{Standard Deviation of } X = S = \sqrt{\frac{\sum_{i=1}^{n}(X_I - \overline{X})^2}{n-1}}$$

The standard error is a measure of the average deviation of *summary statistics* (means, proportions, rates) around their mean assuming infinite repeated sampling:

$$\text{Normal}: \text{s.e.}(\overline{X}) = \frac{S}{\sqrt{n}} = \sqrt{\frac{\frac{\sum_{i=1}^{n}(X_i - \overline{X})^2}{n-1}}{n}}$$

The calculation of standard errors for proportions and rates depends on whether they are in their decimal form, ($0<=p<=1$, $0<=r<=1$), or in their integer form (percents, or per 1,000, 10,000, 100,000 etc.):

$$\text{Binomial}: \text{s.e.}(p) = \sqrt{\frac{p(1-p)}{n}}$$

where p takes on values from 0 to 1

or

$$\text{Binomial}: \text{s.e.}(\%) = \sqrt{\frac{\%(100-\%)}{n}}$$

where % takes on values from 1 to 100

$$\text{Poisson}: \text{s.e.}(r) = \sqrt{\frac{r}{n}}$$

where r takes on values from 0 to 1

or

$$\text{Poisson}: \text{s.e.}(\text{rate}) = \sqrt{\frac{\text{rate}}{n}} \times \text{multiplier}$$

where rate takes on values $>=1$, and multiplier $= 1,000, 10,000, 100,000$

Just as summary statistics (means, proportions, and rates) are all averages and analogous to one another, so too, their standard errors are analogous under certain conditions:

$$\sqrt{\dfrac{\sum\limits_{i=1}^{n}\left(X_i - \overline{X}\right)^2}{n-1}} \cong \sqrt{\dfrac{p(1-p)}{n}} \cong \sqrt{\dfrac{r}{n}}$$

In particular, when an event is very rare (a proportion is very small), the formulas for the binomial and Poisson standard errors are close approximations of one another:

$$\sqrt{\dfrac{p(1-p)}{n}} \cong \sqrt{\dfrac{p(1)}{n}} \cong \sqrt{\dfrac{r}{n}}$$

3.   Measures of Association

Difference Measures:

$$\text{Means}: \overline{X}_1 - \overline{X}_2, \quad \text{Proportions}: p_1 - p_2, \quad \text{Rates}: r_1 - r_2$$

		Outcome		
		Yes	No	
Risk	Yes	a	b	n_1
Factor	No	c	d	n_2
		m_1	m_2	N

$$\dfrac{a}{n_1} - \dfrac{c}{n_2} = p_1 - p_2 \text{ or } r_1 - r_2$$

$$\text{Attributable Risk} = p_1 - p_2$$

$$\text{Population Attributable Risk} = \text{Attributable Risk} \times \text{Prevalence of Risk}$$

$$p_0 - p_2 = (p_1 - p_2) \times \dfrac{n_1}{N}$$

$$\text{Preventive Fraction} = \dfrac{p_2 - p_1}{p_2} = 1 - \text{Relative Risk}$$

Ratio Measures:

$$\text{RR and RP} = \dfrac{\dfrac{a}{a+b}}{\dfrac{c}{c+d}} = \dfrac{\dfrac{a}{n_1}}{\dfrac{c}{n_2}} = \dfrac{r_1}{r_2} \text{ or } \dfrac{p_1}{p_2}$$

Crude:

$$\text{OR} = \dfrac{\dfrac{a}{b}}{\dfrac{c}{d}} = \dfrac{ad}{bc}$$

273

Rothman - Boice Summary Relative Risk :

$$= \frac{\displaystyle\sum_{i=1}^{\# strata} \frac{a_i n_{2i}}{N_i}}{\displaystyle\sum_{i=1}^{\# strata} \frac{c_i n_{1i}}{N_i}}$$

Adjusted:

Mantel - Haenszel Summary Odds Ratio :

$$= \frac{\displaystyle\sum_{i=1}^{\# strata} \frac{a_i d_i}{N_i}}{\displaystyle\sum_{i=1}^{\# strata} \frac{b_i c_i}{N_i}}$$

4. Test Statistics

General form of test statistics:

$$\text{Test Statistic} = \frac{\text{Observed Association - Expected Association}}{\text{Standard Error of the Association}}$$

Test for the Difference Between Two Independent Means:

$$t = \frac{\overline{X}_1 - \overline{X}_2 - 0}{\sqrt{\dfrac{(n_1 - 1)S_1^2 + (n_2 - 1)S_2^2}{n_1 + n_2 - 2}\left(\dfrac{1}{n_1} + \dfrac{1}{n_2}\right)}}$$

where S is the standard deviation of the observed values

Test for the Difference Between Two Independent Proportions or Rates

$$\chi^2 = \sum_{i=a}^{d} \frac{(O_i - E_i)^2}{E_i}$$

where O_i = the observed value in each cell

and $E_i = \dfrac{\text{row total} \times \text{column total}}{N}$

or

$$z = \frac{(p_1 - p_2) - 0}{\sqrt{p_0(1 - p_0)\left(\dfrac{1}{n_1} + \dfrac{1}{n_2}\right)}} \qquad \text{and} \qquad z = \frac{r_1 - r_2 - 0}{\sqrt{r_0\left(\dfrac{1}{n_1} + \dfrac{1}{n_2}\right)}}$$

For the z tests, p_1 and $r_1 = \dfrac{a}{n_1}$, p_2 and $r_2 = \dfrac{c}{n_2}$, and p_0 and $r_0 = \dfrac{m_1}{N}$

Test for Difference Between a Proportion or Rate and a Standard

$$z = \frac{p_1 - \text{Standard}}{\sqrt{\dfrac{\text{Standard}(1 - \text{Standard})}{n_1}}} \quad \text{or} \quad z = \frac{r_1 - \text{Standard}}{\sqrt{\dfrac{\text{Standard}}{n_1}}}$$

Test for the Relative Risk and Relative Prevalence:

$$z = \frac{\ln\left(\dfrac{r_1}{r_2}\right) - 0}{\sqrt{\left(\dfrac{1}{a} \times \dfrac{b}{n_1}\right) + \left(\dfrac{1}{c} \times \dfrac{d}{n_2}\right)}}$$

Test for the Odds Ratio

$$z = \frac{\ln\left(\dfrac{a \times d}{b \times c}\right) - 0}{\sqrt{\dfrac{1}{a} + \dfrac{1}{b} + \dfrac{1}{c} + \dfrac{1}{d}}}$$

5. Confidence Intervals

General form of confidence intervals:

$$CI = \text{Estimate} \pm \text{Critical Value} \times \text{Standard Error of the Estimate}$$

$$CI = \text{Association} \pm \text{Critical Value} \times \text{Standard Error of the Association}$$

Confidence intervals around single estimates:

$$CI(\overline{X}) = \overline{X} \pm 1.96 \frac{S}{\sqrt{n}}$$

$$CI(p) = p \pm 1.96 \sqrt{\frac{p(1-p)}{n}}$$

$$CI(r) = r \pm 1.96 \sqrt{\frac{r}{n}}$$

$$CI(d) = d \pm 1.96 \sqrt{d}$$

where d is a count
of rare health events

Confidence intervals around measures of association:

Difference Measures

$$\text{Normal}: CI = \overline{X}_1 - \overline{X}_2 \pm 1.96 \sqrt{\frac{S_1^2}{n_1} + \frac{S_2^2}{n_2}}$$

$$\text{Binomial}: CI = p_1 - p_2 \pm 1.96 \sqrt{\frac{p_1(1-p_1)}{n_1} + \frac{p_2(1-p_2)}{n_2}}$$

$$\text{Poisson}: CI = r_1 - r_2 \pm 1.96 \sqrt{\frac{r_1}{n_1} + \frac{r_2}{n_2}}$$

Ratio Measures

$$CI_{RR \text{ and } RP} = e^{\left(\ln\left(\frac{r_1}{r_2}\right) \pm 1.96 \sqrt{\left(\frac{1}{a} \times \frac{b}{n_1}\right) + \left(\frac{1}{c} \times \frac{d}{n_2}\right)} \right)}$$

$$CI_{OR} = e^{\left(\ln\left(\frac{a \times d}{b \times c}\right) \pm 1.96 \sqrt{\frac{1}{a} + \frac{1}{b} + \frac{1}{c} + \frac{1}{d}} \right)}$$

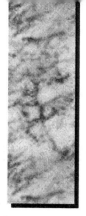

Index

F

Force of Morbidity or Mortality: *see
Incidence Density* 19-20
Funding formulas: *see Resource Allocation*

H

Health Resources and Services
    Administration (HRSA) ix
Hypothesis testing 47-51, 53-56, 61-63,
    104-113, 118-119, 129-130

I

Incidence rates 18-21, 117-118, 128
        Cumulative incidence 19
        Incidence density 19
Index construction 163-167
Information-based decision-making xiii-
    xiv
Integer ranking 147-148, 161

M

Mantel-Haenszel Summary Odds Ratio
    88
Maternal and Child Health Bureau
    (MCHB) ix
Means 12-14, 22-25
Measures of association 48-60, 63-72

N

National Center for Health Statistics
    240-242
Needs assessment x, xiv

O

Odds Ratio (OR) 63-70, 108-113, 125-127,
    133-134
Omnibus Budget Reconciliation Act
    (OBRA) 1989 ix, x

P

Percentile rescaling 148-152, 161
Planning cycle xiv
Population Attributable Risk (PAR) 57-
    60

Population Attributable Risk
    percent 59-60
Prevalence rates 18, 116-118, 128
Preventive fraction 71, 119, 130
Probability distribution 32-34, 38
        Normal 32, 35, 39
        Binomial 32, 34, 35
        Poisson 32, 34, 35
        Chi-square 32, 33
        F 32, 33
        Exponential 32
Program evaluation xiv, 81-85
Proportions 12-14, 15, 34-38, 50-56, 61-
    63

R

Ranking: *see Integer Ranking*
Rates 15-21, 34-38, 61-63, 115-116, 127
Ratios 15, 63
Regression methods 104-113, 125-127,
    133-134
        Logistic 104, 108-112
        Ordinary Least Squares (OLS)
            104, 105-108, 209-210
        Poisson 104, 211-212
Relative Prevalence (RP) 63-70
Relative Risk (RR) 63-70, 99, 100
        Adjusted Relative Risk 87, 92-94
        Rothman-Boice Summary
        Relative Risk 87
Resource allocation 168-172
Risk factor v. risk marker 5

S

Sampling 29-32
Scoring: *see Integer Ranking, Percentile
Rescaling, z-scores, z-tests*
Standard deviation 35
Standardization of Rates 92-100
        Direct 95, 98-100
        Indirect 95-100
Study Designs 77-85
        Intervention Studies 81
        Observational Studies 81
        Experimental Designs 81, 82
Quasi-Experimental Designs 81, 82